Man Trap

First published in 2008 by
Liberties Press
Guinness Enterprise Centre | Taylor's Lane | Dublin 8
Tel: +353 (1) 415 1224
www.LibertiesPress.com | info@libertiespress.com

Distributed in the United States by
Dufour Editions | PO Box 7 | Chester Springs | Pennsylvania | 19425

and in Australia by
James Bennett Pty Limited | InBooks | 3 Narabang Way
Belrose NSW 2085

Trade enquiries to CMD Distribution
55A Spruce Avenue | Stillorgan Industrial Park
Blackrock | County Dublin
Tel: +353 (1) 294 2560 | Fax: +353 (1) 294 2564

ISBN: 978–1–905483–56–3
2 4 6 8 10 9 7 5 3 1

A CIP record for this title is available from the British Library.

Cover design by Siné Design
Internal design by Liberties Press
Printed in Ireland by Colour Books | Baldoyle Industrial Estate | Dublin 13

Man Trap

Dealing with Prostate Cancer

The Irish Story

Rory Hafford

By the same author

Killing the Magpie:
The Search for Health and Happiness

For Catherine,
Sam and Katie

Contents

Acknowledgements

To all my friends and colleagues in Carr Communications who read the manuscript and supported me throughout this project. To the doctors who gave me the benefit of their time and expertise. To the patients whose stories illuminated the text. To Ruben, for all the work he put into the early design. To Peter and Sean at Liberties, who had the bravery to run with the project in the first place and whose skill and know-how made it a much better book in the end. To John B. Keane, who set the ball rolling.

Introduction

Time Bombs

From the moment we are born, genetically we are programmed to die . . .

It was during this delicate programming stage that tiny biological incendiary bombs were factored into our make-up, hidden in corners, tucked away in folds; ticking slowly, insidiously, inexorably.

Millions of years from now, when the old super-race lands on Earth and starts sifting through the biological debris that was mankind, they will stumble upon the prostate and ask: 'Was this the thing that led to the obliteration of the human race?'

And, at least for the thousands of men who are diagnosed with, and succumb to, prostate cancer every year, you could make the case that it was.

For them, the time-bomb not only ticked away all their life – it went off!

It's time for a new focus.

Every few weeks, it appears, books are written about the problem of breast

9

cancer, cervical cancer and osteoporosis - conditions and diseases that are peculiar to women. And this is as it should be.

For the longest time, women have been proactive about their own health and have been supported in their endeavours by health legislators, focus groups and the pharmaceutical industry when it comes to demanding better health care.

And this is also as it should be.

However, health care should not be a gender issue; brother should not be set against sister in this matter. Health care should be apportioned in equal measure because 'We are all equal'. Right? Sadly, this is not the case.

Men are not particularly vigorous about fighting their own corner when it comes to looking after their health. Men are more inclined to ignore health problems than to face up to them. Men are more likely to die from diseases that are preventable.

One of these diseases is prostate cancer - a condition that has stepped up its deadly march in recent years. The number of Irish men diagnosed each and every year with prostate cancer has nearly doubled since the mid-1990s. The number of Irish men dying from this disease is also on the increase, and now stands at between 500 and 600 a year. The tragedy of this situation lies in the fact that prostate cancer is like any other cancer, in that if you catch it early you have a much better chance of successfully treating the disease.

So, it could be argued, it would make sense to look for this condition, or to screen for it early. Yet we don't have a screening programme in this country for prostate cancer.

We have a breast cancer screening programme; we have just introduced a cervical cancer screening programme. But no prostate screening programme. And no plans for one.

Every day, it appears, women are telling their story. But men have a story to tell as well. And our story begins in a little country town on the south-west coast of Ireland.

1

John B.

The tiny Kerry town of Listowel is shining like a bright new button. The heavy, dark clouds that had earlier frowned down upon the picture-postcard streets had blown away out to sea, and a blindingly blue sky took its place centre stage. If ever there was a day when it was 'good to be alive', this was it.

The RTÉ health crew was in town to shoot a documentary on poet, raconteur, wit, publican and all-round fabulous human being, John B. Keane.

His little pub opened up to us like a mother's hug. Warm, snug, welcoming.

John B. was perched on a bar stool, reading a well-thumbed copy of the *Kerryman*.

As the camera crew began clattering around, looking for the 'place with the best light' and the best 'angles', and alcoves that would help the sound to 'bounce', John B. snapped into inimitable action.

Reading loudly from his newspaper, an exaggerated Kerry accent coming back off the walls, he joked: 'The local Kerry magistrate has issued a writ for two decidedly dodgy-looking characters – one carrying a camera, the other struggling under the weight of a giant boom.'

The whimsy was typical of the man. Wherever John B. saw humour, he had to give voice to it. Whenever he could bring laughter to a situation, he simply couldn't help himself. Wherever there was life, he would live it.

That was why it was with a heavy heart that we went to Listowel to interview John B. on one specific issue: prostate cancer.

He had been diagnosed with the disease just a few months prior to our arrival and, like most men, was struggling to come to terms with the dreadful ramifications of the diagnosis.

He wanted to talk about it. His doctor wanted him to talk about it. The doctor felt that if John B. brought the issue out into the open, if he could in some way highlight it, it might encourage more men to take better care of themselves.

The playwright wanted to talk, but he wasn't sure what to say. For the first time in his life, words seemed to be failing him. There were so many conflicting issues, and all of them were juggling for space in his tortured mind: Why him? Why this form of cancer? Why couldn't it have been caught earlier? Would his treatment regime work? How long did he have? So many questions; so few direct answers.

When the camera started to roll, John B. gathered himself and switched to type. The positive man began to emerge, the storyteller, the people-pleaser.

In short, he did his job. He did what people expected of him.

He told people that there was a gland called the prostate. He told people that, in some men, it had a tendency to turn cancerous. He told people where to go if they had any further questions or concerns.

But when the camera was switched off, that's when the real story emerged. The story of how he had to wear nappies to his daughter's wedding. The story of how he lay awake at night in a panic. The story of not knowing whether his treatment would work.

Afterwards, as we shared a drink alone away in a corner, his expression changed and became dark. Like sun disappearing off a field.

He kept asking one question. Just one: 'Why couldn't they have caught this horrible thing sooner?'

A couple of years after the story aired on RTÉ television, John B. Keane passed away. The fight had drained him. The playwright always knew when it was time for the curtain to fall. It was time.

For the sake of John B. Keane, for the sake of the hundreds of Irish men who will die as a result of prostate cancer this year, we are going to ask this question again and again until we get an answer that makes sense: *Why don't we have a prostate cancer screening programme?*

2

Screen Saver

Florence. The Piazza della Signoria. A group of leading Irish travel-health doctors are whiling away the hours under a velvet-blue night sky and toasting Italian hospitality.

The event is the European Travel Medicine Conference. The great and the good are gathered to discuss such tantalising topics as dengue fever, the Ebola virus and the rampant spread of HIV.

It is hardly the forum for prostate cancer. But nonetheless, the topic is broached. Opinions are, predictably, divided. Some of the older doctors feel that there is not enough hard evidence to suggest that current test criteria warrant a full-scale screening programme for Ireland. Other doctors, particularly the younger ones, feel that the issue is not one of screening but one of control!

'Listen,' said one doctor, a young GP with a burgeoning practice in Cork, 'if you look for something, you have a better chance of finding it. That, for men, is the bottom line.'

Fair enough. But what if a man in the prostate 'at risk' group presented to him with something as innocuous as a throat infection? Would he screen him for prostate cancer as a matter of course?

'No, because the onus shouldn't be on me to screen for prostate cancer. There should be a programme in place where it happens as a matter of course and the efforts of GPs are acknowledged and rewarded accordingly.'

OK. What if a man in the 'at risk' group asked to be screened?

'They wouldn't. Most men are inherently weak at asking for medical help, and this is with problems that they are currently suffering with, let alone something that only *might* happen in the future. Men don't ask for help. It's not in their make-up.'

Another doctor, sipping on a Bacardi Breezer and listening intently, was even more direct about what he perceived as the lack of action on the screening front: 'This is all about money. The people who control the purse strings in the Department of Health simply don't want to invest in stemming what is a small tide of prostate-cancer cases. They feel the money would be better spent elsewhere.'

And he didn't stop there. 'Also, the lack of urologists [specialists who treat

prostate problems, among other condi-
tions] in Ireland is an outrage. And as
far as I am aware, we are some way away
from bringing this number up to an accept-
able level. You could be forgiven for
thinking that the inactivity in this area
is down to control: the fewer urologists
there are, the more work they have – for
themselves!'

Intriguing. The problem, on face value,
is not as clear-cut as it first appeared.
Even the usual massed ranks of the medical
profession seem bitterly divided on the
issue.

Time for a bit of old-fashioned jour-
nalistic investigation . . .

Better Days

Hawkins House, the home of the Department
of Health, has seen better days. Located
right in the middle of Dublin city centre,
the building itself is in need of major
refurbishment. Some would argue, perhaps
unkindly, that the building mirrors the
state of the health service generally:
that is, in need of more than just a lick
of paint. In the great prostate debate,
it's my first port of call.

Armed with a series of basic questions,
I approach the Department's communications office with a request for inter-
views. None are forthcoming. I protest. To
no avail. I decide to fax in my list to
the press office:

§ Why don't we have a prostate screening programme in Ireland?

§ Are we going to see an increase in the number of urologists to tackle the rise in prostate cases?

§ What advice are you giving to 'at risk' men?

§ If you have a BreastCheck screening service for women to detect cancers peculiar to women, why not a screening service to detect cancers peculiar to men?

Here's what I got back. It turns out that prostate cancer is part of a bigger picture that takes in the whole area of medical screening. That's the good news. The bad news is that one of the biggest cancer killers of men in this country is not considered high enough priority to have even its own specialised committee.

'As part of the work being undertaken by the National Cancer Forum, a subgroup was established on generic screening,' said the department's reply. 'This multidisciplinary group has reviewed all issues relating to screening, including examining specific diseases such as prostate and colorectal cancer. In relation to screening for prostate in particular, the group recommended that there is currently insufficient evidence to recommend the introduction of a population-based prostate screening programme in this country.'

The statement continued: 'The Group recommends that this issue should be reassessed when the results are available from randomised trials currently being conducted.'

Regarding the paucity of urologists, the department is looking closely at the issue: 'The Report of the National Task Force on Medical Staffing recommended that the number of consultant urologists be increased by over 100 percent, from twenty-three to forty-nine posts by the year 2009. The Task Force concluded that this increase would "meet the require-ments of the European Working Time Directive to achieve a consultant-provid-ed service and ensure high standards in medical education and training".

'A key consideration in increasing the number of consultant posts was whether there would be a sufficient, suitably com-plex workload available to individual consultants to ensure that they main-tained expertise and met audit and accred-itation criteria. A sufficient critical mass of workload is also necessary to support the provision of satisfactory medical education and training.'

Cutting Edge

That was the official line of the Department of Health, the people charged with looking after our health and wellbeing. Let's pick over the bones of what they said - because somebody has to, just to make sense of it!

It is recommended that the number of urologists be increased, with the proviso that there has to be enough work to 'keep them going', as it were.

Around 600 Irish men are dying every year from prostate cancer. It begs the question: 'Is that enough work for you, fellas?'

They also say that there is insufficient evidence to support the introduction of a prostate screening programme in Ireland. Let's put this issue to bed, once and for all.

Professor John Fitzpatrick - a man who works at the leading edge of prostate-cancer research in this country - has called for a screening programme to be considered. Or, if not a full-blown screening programme, at least a dedicated Irish study to check out the viability of one.

Professor Fred Stephens of the University of Sydney is also an expert in the area of prostate cancer. He is on record as saying: 'The earlier a patient seeks medical attention for anything unusual or different, the more likely it will be that any cancer will be detected at a curable stage.'

He continues: 'If any cancer is detected early, while it is still small and before it has spread to another place, it can usually be completely removed surgically, or destroyed in some other way, so that its eradication or cure can be achieved before any serious damage has been done. If these early cancers are completely removed before they have spread, their danger will have been eliminated and the patient will be cured. This is as true of prostate cancer as any other type of cancer.'

Hold on. That's worth repeating: *'This is as true of prostate cancer as any other type of cancer.'*

Dr Patrick Walsh of the world-famous Johns Hopkins Hospital in Baltimore, Maryland, is also spreading a pro-screening message. 'Since screening came in, fewer men present with a cancer that has spread. More men present with curable disease. More men are being offered curable therapy, and deaths from prostate cancer in the US have fallen by 30 percent,' says Dr Walsh.

Dr Andrew von Eschenbach of the National Cancer Institute in the US is another advocate of catching this disease at an early stage. He says: 'Our best weapon today to deal with cancer is to be able to find it early, at a time when we can still effectively apply treatment.'

In America, pro-screening forces would appear to be winning the argument. At least twenty-six states have already passed laws mandating that health insurers include Prostate Specific Antigen (PSA) tests (which are designed to test for activity in the prostate) in the policies they sell consumers. Medical analysts believe that the high-profile prostate cancers, such as those that affected 'Stormin' Norman Schwarzkopf, are likely to renew widespread calls for screening to be made compulsory.

OK, so we're beginning to get a picture of the politics of prostate cancer. And it's a murky one.

Now, let's put a face on the condition itself. What is this killer of men?

3

My Mate Jack

Mention the word 'prostate', and a number of questions usually spring to mind. Chief among them are: The prostate! What's that, then? Where does it reside? Why do we need one in the first place?

The irony is that we only seem to focus on this little gland when it becomes a big problem.

OK, here's the science bit. The prostate is a tiny gland that is peculiar to men. Size-wise, it is about the same as a walnut, or a golf ball. Where it is located has a lot to do with its function.

Root around for a while, and you are sure to come across it somewhere between the bladder and the rectum. (Now that I think of it, I don't believe I will root around for it!)

What's a gland? A gland is a tiny organ that secretes chemical substances. To this end, the prostate makes and stores a special fluid that is an essential part of semen, and this fluid is released during ejaculation. (OK, I'm *definitely* not rooting around for it!)

There was a time, however, when I did spend a few weeks rooting around for the prostate. The thing is, it wasn't *my* prostate . . .

I was part of a motley crew of medical-science students who were assigned our own cadaver. We were instructed to treat the 'body that had been left to science' with the utmost respect and dignity at all times; an edict we observed rigorously – with one exception.

We dubbed the guy 'Jack', because we were slap-bang in the middle of Ireland's amazing Italia '90 World Cup run under the canny eye of the big Geordie, Jack Charlton. At one point, when 'The Bhoys in Green' beat England, courtesy of a deft header from Ray Houghton, someone stuck a green-and-white-hooped bobbin hat on our cadaver. It stayed there for the duration of the team's World Cup run.

I got to know our 'Jack' pretty well. Some would say too well. We were all assigned different areas of the body. I got the reproductive system. Pulling and dragging away at folds of skin and what seemed like miles of tubing is not the most pleasurable way to pass the time. And Jack's system was particularly hard to navigate. It was a bit like hacking your way through an overgrown rainforest. It would have helped to know where you were going in the first place. We didn't. When you are starting out, there are no sign-posts to help you on your way. You recog-nise nothing. It's trial, error and even more error.

My destination was the prostate. My mission, should I choose to accept it, was to get in, lay it bare and 'describe its gross anatomy'. Gross!

'OK,' announced our anatomy professor, in a voice that bounced back off antisep-tic walls, 'all you students on the repro-ductive system need to be aware of a few landmarks, namely: the *corpus cavernosum* [that's the erectile tissue to meself and yourself], the urethra, the spermatic cord and the epididymis.'

A small, burly man, very much in the mode of Danny DeVito, he paused briefly for effect. And then continued: 'Once you have found these, I want you to work your way into the area of the prostate.'

'Feel for it,' he said, his hands put-ting on a play in front of him, squeezing little pockets of air. 'It will feel a little like a spongy mass. The potential urologists in the group will be able to tell if there are signs of cancer in the gland.'

It was the first time I had heard the term 'prostate cancer'. It was not to be the last.

Trouble Brewing

The prostate gland plays a key role in the male reproductive system, secreting a lot of the liquid that the body uses in semen. (During ejaculation, semen is secreted by the prostate through small pores in the walls of the urethra, the tube that carries urine from the bladder.) The prostate is located just beneath the bladder, where it encircles the urethra, a bit like a doughnut.

OK, so we're beginning to get a picture of what this thing does. Now, what does it look like?

Snipping our way through Jack's gnarly folds and tough tubing, we eventually arrived, like jaded jungle explorers, at our destination: the prostate. The site of so much trouble for so many men.

It's made up of three lobes, encased in an outer covering, or capsule. It's a little bit spongy to the touch, although, in Jack's case, it had lost a lot of its characteristic elasticity. It is flanked on either side by the seminal vesicles, a pair of pouch-like glands that stand like two noble soldiers guarding an entranceway to great treasures. The glands themselves contribute to these treasures by adding to the quality of the semen.

Next to the vesicles runs the vas deferens, which consists of tough little tubes that look a bit like train tracks.

Their job is to transport sperm from the epididymis into the ejaculatory duct.

Somewhere deep within the machinery is a switch. Sometimes, somehow, the switch is flipped, and a train of events is set in motion that can lead to prostate cancer.

Although there are several known risk factors for developing prostate cancer, no one knows for sure why one man contracts the disease and another does not. It's a deadly mystery. We have some clues: age plays a part, as do ethnicity, genetics and diet. Age is the big one.

The incidence of prostate cancer rises sharply after the age of sixty – and the majority of men will have some form of prostate 'activity' after the age of eighty. Many will die with the disease, but not because of it. This is an important factor, because it can justifiably allow health 'watchdogs' to do nothing to address the actual cancer. Health professionals have a name for this: they call it 'watchful waiting'. So, in many instances, they do nothing – except watch and wait. But here's the thing: if you wait for something to take hold and do nothing to prevent it, usually it will oblige.

Doctors will argue this with you. They will say – again, justifiably – that because prostate cancer is likely to develop in most men, it can be classed as a 'microscopic disease'. This means that it will not shorten life expectancy, because the cancer takes a long time to grow and to become what the medical profession calls 'clinically important'.

The flip side of this particular coin is that some prostate cancers can take hold quickly, they can develop quickly, and they can spread quickly. There is no template. At no point can the guard be lowered. Ever.

'Jack' was sixty-five when he died. Ironically, there was some evidence of prostate cancer: I could feel little bumps and nodules in the gland. He didn't die because of it, however. In fact, he succumbed to a heart attack.

When he passed away, he was decidedly overweight. So it might be logical to assume that his diet had something to do with his heart problem and the development of some cancer in his prostate.

Food Factors

There is some evidence that a man's diet can influence his risk of developing prostate cancer. The most common dietary culprit in raising the risk is a full-fat menu, particularly a diet high in animal fats. Also, there have recently been a few studies which would seem to suggest that a diet low in vegetables causes an increased risk of developing prostate cancer.

There are a few foods that scientists feel can decrease the risk of developing

cancer of the prostate. These include
tomatoes (or, more specifically, their
lycopene component) and a goodly helping
of omega-3 fatty acids (oils that are
found in fish like salmon and mackerel).
A diet high in selenium and vitamin D is
also thought to be beneficial.

Genetically, Jack didn't fall into a
neat category. His father also died of a
heart attack. He had no brothers, so there
was no pattern of prostate cancer in his
family. However, it is thought that a family history of prostate cancer increases
a man's chances of developing the disease.

So, let's break it down: the increased
risk shows itself when a man has either a
father or brother (or both) who have had
prostate cancer. This risk is even greater
when the cancer develops at an early age
in his relatives.

A number of different genetic factors
are currently being looked at. Men who
carry mutations in genes known as BRCA1 or
BRCA2 may have a two- to five-fold
increase in prostate-cancer risk.
Ironically, these are also the same genes
implicated in breast and ovarian cancer in
women. Men with high levels of testosterone are also thought to be at a higher risk of developing the condition.

'So, what did you find?' asked the
anatomy professor, suddenly hovering on
tippy-toes next to the dissecting table.

'Well, there was some evidence of mod-
ular development in the prostate itself,'
I said, desperately trying to sound as

though I knew what I was talking about. 'I'd say, had he lived a little longer, he would have experienced some metastasis [cancer spread].'

The professor moved in closer still to get a better view of the sizeable cavity that had been gouged in the poor man's lower abdomen. 'Yep,' he said, 'we'll make a pathologist out of you yet.'

He started to leave, stopped himself, and turned back again. 'You do know, however, that a man of that age was bound to develop prostate cancer to some degree. Once you hit sixty, the risk increases considerably.'

However, sometimes it doesn't wait that long . . .

4

Age-old Problem

Most men, if they live long enough, will develop prostate problems.

Strangely enough, this statement is potentially somewhat reassuring as well as terrifying. For some men, particularly the younger ones, it means that they don't have to worry about the prospect of developing a killer disease until they are in their sixties, or their seventies, or even their eighties, should they live that long. It is something that may happen in the dim and distant future.

Right? Wrong!

If it's inevitable that it is going to happen in the future (and all the studies point to this fact), then it has to have a beginning. Burying our head in the sand on the issue means that we are losing out on catching it and treating it in the early stages, when most cancers can be tackled effectively.

But try telling that to a young man in his twenties. For him, cancer is not even a blip on the radar.

Mulligan's pub, just off Dublin's quays area, is a heaving mass. The Guinness is flowing and the craic is ninety!

There is mostly a younger clientele in on this particular Saturday night. The plan is to 'get a few in' and then head off to a nightclub somewhere in the city. Sure, you could end up anywhere. And that's half the fun!

In a bid to ride the wave of alcohol-induced jocularity, I sally forth with an impromptu vox pop. There's a gathering of younger men over in one corner. I move in.

'Hey, fellas! Do you mind if I ask you a couple of questions?'

They look at me quizzically. 'Questions?' asks one, his eyes like daggers. 'What are you, a bleedin' cop or something?'

I figure maybe I should have done a little more research on this whole impromptu-vox-pop thing. 'A cop? Nah, nothing like that. I'm a scientist, actually.'

'You don't look like a fuckin' scientist to me,' says another. 'You look more like a cop.'

'Well, I *am* a scientist, and I'd just like to ask you a couple of questions on prostate cancer . . . if that's OK with you guys.'

'Jesus, dude, you could have picked a better time,' says one. 'We're supposed to be having a bit of fun here. Talk about killing the mood.'

I move to leave.

'Oh, go on then,' says another, catching me before I turn. He looks at his watch and makes a bored face.

I pull up a chair. 'OK. Anyone know what the prostate is?'

'Yeah,' snaps one of the group, a bloke with moppish Gilbert O'Sullivan hair and a mouthful of gleaming white teeth. 'It's a country where hookers rule!'

'No,' says his mate, 'that's a *Pro* State. Scientist Boy here is talking about something else entirely.'

The exchange is greeted with a few high fives and some raucous laughter. I feel like a prick and decide to call it a night before it can get any worse. But as I start to get up off my chair, I feel a hand on my shoulder. 'Yeah, I know what the prostate is.'

I turn to look up into the face of a guy who couldn't be more than twenty.

'I know what it is,' he says, his face turning serious, 'because my dad died from it.'

Clinically Silent

This is usually the circuitous route by which young men come across the issue of prostate cancer: someone close to them develops it.

35

But prostate cancer is no longer the private and tragic domain of the elderly gentleman, as was once believed. True, some 30 percent of men over the age of fifty will have what doctors call 'clinically silent' prostate cancer – and this proportion rises to more than 50 percent in men over eighty. However, the incidence of younger men with the condition is also increasing.

Professor John Fitzpatrick, a prostate expert attached to the Mater Hospital in Dublin, has had men in their thirties present to him with the disease. He wants to get the message out that prostate cancer is not age-specific any more; all men should be aware of the risks.

Professor Mel Greaves, a cell-biology expert at the Institute of Cancer Research in London, says that the first signs of prostate cancer can be spotted very early on. 'In one study,' he says, 'low-grade neoplastic lesions [the precursor to carcinoma] were found in men in their twenties. This suggests that the evolution of prostate cancer can be initiated very early on – and that the natural history of this cancer can be very protracted.'

He suggests another link that may be of interest to younger men: 'Several studies, but not all, have linked prostate cancer with (prior) increased sexual activity in terms of number of partners, frequency of coitus, a history of venereal disease, or desiring more sex than is available.'

We can target the at-risk profile a little more accurately, however. Dr Christopher Dolinsky of the University of Pennsylvania Medical School says that every man over the age of forty-five is at risk of prostate cancer. 'Although prostate cancer can strike younger men, the risk of getting the disease increases with age,' he says. 'More than 70 percent of men diagnosed with prostate cancer are over the age of sixty-five.'

Age is generally considered the most important risk factor for prostate cancer. The incidence of the disease rises quickly after the age of sixty – and the majority of men will have some form of prostate cancer after the age of eighty.

But let's backtrack a little and pay a visit to Professor Fitzpatrick's place . . .

5

The Heart Says Yes!

To describe Professor John Fitzpatrick as simply a urologist is a bit like calling Pelé just another footballer. The good professor is at the top of his profession. When he talks, people listen.

He has been talking about prostate screening for some time. Let's listen to him: 'For too long now, people have linked prostate cancer to an aged population. This is wrong. Certainly, it's a condition that presents more often in older men, but not exclusively. There are widespread cases of men in their early fifties being diagnosed with prostate cancer. There are cases of men in their forties being diagnosed with prostate cancer. I myself have had men in my surgery, Irish men in their thirties, who have shown signs of activity in the prostate. It is a condition that all men should be concerned about.'

It is a condition that all men should be concerned about!

Professor Fitzpatrick practises out of rooms on Dublin's Eccles Street, just across from the impressive stone-pillared façade that is the front entrance of the Mater Hospital.

He himself is physically impressive too. He stands over six feet tall; he is always impeccably dressed, usually in an understated pinstripe suit; he sports a shock of wavy steel-grey hair; when he engages with you, he locks on.

He is also impressive to listen to. His voice has a rich, melodic quality to it; when he talks, the information – hard to take though some of it might be – gently washes over you. You get the impression that it is a well-practised timbre, designed in no small measure to ease troubled hearts and tortured minds. That said, it could also be very much just a mark of the man.

Professor Fitzpatrick is well versed on the PSA/prostate debate. Well versed, and very balanced.

'There are two sides to the screening story,' he says. 'PSA testing was introduced in 1989 by the FDA [the US Food and Drug Administration] as a way to monitor the disease, not as an actual screening tool.

'A few years after that [in 1991], a paper was published in the *New England Journal of Medicine* which stated that screening was definitely the way forward on prostate cancer. On publication of that paper, the FDA took the step of announcing that PSA should be used as a screening tool. But PSA, on its own, was never designed for this purpose, and I don't believe it was up to the challenge.'

I detect a slight swing in the professor's direction. A few years before, as part of a special RTÉ documentary on prostate cancer, he was fairly vocal in calling for a new focus on screening. Now, he is less so. Now, he is sticking very much to the evidence; taking baby steps instead of giant strides forward.

Simple Logic

Part of me feels let down. Part of me feels that he has lost the will to continue to fight on this issue. Dealing with the bureaucrats can wear you down over the years, like waves against a rock face: eventually, your edge begins to blunt. Maybe he's tired. Maybe he's just taking a break. But then again, if someone as influential as Professor John Fitzpatrick is beginning to wane, what hope is there?

I persist with my simple logic. What about breast-cancer screening, I ask him. Doesn't this initiative, which addresses a problem particular to women, show the way forward for an exclusively male ailment?

'There is no doubt that breast-cancer screening has shown the way forward in this regard. However, even though prostate cancer is such a huge killer of men in this country, it doesn't necessarily follow that we should adopt the same approach. We need conclusive evidence which will allow us to progress on this issue.'

Evidence! I want to scream! Evidence takes resources and money, and we don't have any. Anyway, isn't there enough evidence from trials in other countries? Evidence also takes time to accumulate, and we are all out of time. Men are dying now. Hundreds will die this year alone. We need action, and we need it now!

But I don't have to scream anything at the man. He knows.

Suddenly, he changes. His mood, his tone: everything shifts.

'Look,' he says, 'it's all very well for the government to say they won't move forward on screening until they have hard evidence. But screening, after a fashion, is already happening. All over Ireland there is back-door screening being carried out. Men are going to their GP and are asking for tests to be done. So, you could argue, screening is already taking place.

'What the government needs to do now is show some initiative and pull this piecemeal approach together and put their weight behind a real screening study. We need to organise this into a trial.'

That's more like it! That's the professor I remember from the RTÉ documentary. And he's not finished; he is also deeply unhappy about the dearth of urologists in Ireland.

'The lack of urologists in this country is nothing short of a disgrace! When it comes to urologist cover, we are the lowest in Europe by head of population, and this situation cannot be allowed to continue. The number of urologists in this country needs to be doubled – and the government needs to address this problem now.'

When he is finished, I feel I can detect just a faint hint of sulphur in the air. He visibly calms himself, and begins to pull the strands of our conversation together.

'On a national screening programme for prostate cancer, my heart says yes. I do believe that we need to diagnose this disease early to give ourselves the best chance of treating it effectively. I know that screening is available in many areas of the States, for instance. But I also believe that we need an Irish study to give us Irish evidence so that we can tailor a programme specifically for this country.'

Outside, the rain is beginning to fall, pounding the pavement. Across the way, a middle-aged man is helped from a cab. He is ushered slowly up the steps of the Mater Hospital under the protection of a black umbrella that has seen better days.

I wonder what he has. I wonder if they've caught it in time.

6

The Flip Side

'Prostate screening is a nightmare issue. There is nothing black and white about it . . . '

I'm talking to Dr Hugh Gallagher, one of Ireland's leading urologists, and a man who has very definite views on the whole prostate debate.

I sense that he is not that comfortable talking to me. I sense that he doesn't really want to be seen to come down on one particular side of the fence.

'Prostate screening is multifaceted. There is no right or wrong answer,' he says, just a touch of angst in his voice.

He is fully aware of the human face of this disease. Every day, he sees the physical and psychological torment caused by a condition that suddenly springs its horrible surprise on a small army of unsuspecting men.

He agrees fully that if you look for something, you have a better chance of finding it. He agrees absolutely that prostate cancer is like every other cancer, in that if you catch it early, you have a better chance of treating it effectively.

However, he feels that we still have to stick to the facts on this issue. 'Either we follow the laws of evidence-based medicine, or we don't. As doctors, we have to work with the most up-to-date information and the published studies. At the moment, the evidence seems to be pointing to the fact that screening on a nationwide basis is not the way to go.'

I push him on this: why not?

He gathers himself. You can see him weighing the options in his head. For a second, intellect and emotion collide. Intellect is winning the struggle. He cites a recent European study which found that 4 percent of men between the ages of forty and seventy-five had some form of prostate cancer.

'If you extrapolate these figures down to an Irish context, that's about 400,000 Irish men. Now, 4 percent of that total represents between 13,000 and 18,000 [men] who need urgent prostate care. Break those figures down even further and you have in the region of 750 patients for every urologist in Ireland.

'It's simply unworkable. It would mean that if we worked flat out we would still only be able to deal with the prostate patients, and every other urological problem would go by the wayside.'

This is probably the best argument we have heard so far to increase radically the number of urologists in this country.

Screening is one thing. Dr Gallagher is also very concerned about what happens when you *do* uncover something. 'Some of what we have to do is very radical. Some of the side effects can be equally as radical, leading to things like erectile dysfunction and incontinence. In a younger man, this is not just an inconvenience, it's completely life-altering. In some ways, it's life-destroying.'

In his book *What To Do When They Say It's Cancer*, counsellor Joel Nathan addresses the issue of the loss of sexual power as a result of prostate cancer from the point of view of the emotions. He says that sexual potency makes an interesting marker of 'quality of life', for men at least.

'Aware that sexuality is intimately linked to our life-force, the authors of one study focused on discovering how men would respond to the choice between survival on one hand and maintaining sexual potency on the other, if they underwent surgery for prostate cancer,' writes Nathan.

'The basis of the trial was that while surgery for prostate cancer offers a higher survival rate (90 percent at five years), it also produces a 90–100 percent rate of sexual impotency. Radiotherapy,

the alternative, produces a 20–50 percent
rate of impotency, but the survival rate
is much lower.'

It all comes down to a question of
choice . . .

'Patients should be permitted to choose
medical treatments according to their own
values, beliefs, preferences and life-
goals,' says Nathan. 'In this way,
patients are empowered to put into operation the concept of autonomy. People can
exercise this right to choose only if
their physician informs them of options in
treatments.'

In short, decisions have to be made.
But who is going to help Irish men make
those decisions?

7

Zero Tolerance

The Political Approach

Abbey Street in Dublin's city centre is moving at a crawl. Queues are long and tempers are short.

It's coming up to 'quitting time', and people are trying to steal a march on the crowds, but to no avail. It seems that, no matter what time of the day or night, Dublin is in gridlock.

The authorities, in fairness to them, have racked their brains in a bid to solve the traffic problem. Basically, as far as we can make out, their 'solution' consists of a two-pronged approach:

1.   demonise the motorist;

2.   criminalise the motorist.

Outside the old offices of Independent Newspapers, an unfortunate woman is going through the indignity of having her car clamped. She is pleading and begging with the clamper, who, it appears, couldn't be more uninterested in her plight.

'I'm only five minutes over my time,' she tries to reason, her face a mask of pure angst.

'Sorry, missus,' says the clamper. 'As far as I'm concerned you are illegally parked. That means you are breaking the law.'

He turns to look at her, apparently softening for a second: 'Listen, I don't make the rules, I only enforce them.'

Welcome to modern-day Ireland. A place where rule, regulation, red tape and road rage abound. A place where zero tolerance is not just a slogan, it's an unfortunate way of life. A place where, if you think or step outside the box, you are hammered by 'due process'. A place where there is no longer any wiggle room.

In time, zero tolerance can, it has been argued, turn people into virtual robots, mechanically – and fearfully – moving from box to box in ever-decreasing circles.

Medicine, in Ireland, is now practised in exactly the same way. Evidence-based medicine is a form of zero tolerance: show me the proof, and then – and only then – will we act.

The issue of prostate screening is treated in exactly this way here. The people who make the decisions on population-based health care have decided that the 'risks' of screening for prostate cancer outweigh the benefits.

They have decided that the economic costs, the potential psychological fall-out, and the possible physical side effects need further investigation before they will even think about an alternative approach.

One of the big arguments for not introducing a screening programme lies in the fact that the unfortunately named Prostate Specific Antigen test is not specific enough. An elevated PSA reading does not necessarily mean that the patient has prostate cancer. It could mean a whole host of other things instead, like that he has a simple bladder infection, for instance.

What's needed is a much more sensitive test. Well, it just so happens . . .

C Change

The flash Four Seasons Hotel in Dublin's very leafy, and very exclusive, Ballsbridge was the scene for a recent – and hugely important – medical conference. It was important for one main reason: it presented a potential way forward out of the current morass that is prostate-testing options.

It was addressed by Mr John Thornhill, a consultant urologist of worldwide renown.

49

But let's look at the facts before we look at the findings from this conference. We currently have a test called a PSA, which works by indicating 'activity' in the prostate gland. The medical profession is not particularly happy with this test because, for one thing, it is felt that the test is not conclusive enough.

An elevated PSA reading could point to the early development of prostate cancer, certainly. Alternatively, it could also point to something as simple as a urinary-tract infection. Therefore, a doctor is loath to order a fully battery of tests, which could include a biopsy of the prostate itself, based only on an elevated PSA reading.

The good news from the Four Seasons conference comes in the form of a new prostate test. It's called a cPSA, or complex PSA. Strictly speaking, it's not that new. It has been around for a number of years, but only now are the test results of this procedure coming back – and they are very encouraging.

cPSA makes the diagnostic process that little bit more accurate and effective and gives the zero-tolerance brigade a little bit more to think about.

Trial Run

Further testing to advance the sensitivity of the PSA process is taking place in the US, primarily through a programme known as the PLCO trial. Here's just a brief sample of some of the methods being studied:

PSA velocity

This is based on changes in PSA levels over time. A sharp rise in the level increases the suspicion of cancer.

Age-adjusted PSA

Age is an important factor in increasing PSA levels, as we have seen. For this reason, some doctors use age-adjusted PSA readings to determine when diagnostic tests are needed. When age-adjusted PSA levels are used, a different PSA level is defined as normal for each ten-year age group. Doctors who use this method generally suggest that men younger than fifty should have a PSA reading below 2.4 ng/ml, while a PSA level up to 6.5 ng/ml would be considered normal for men in their seventies. Doctors currently do not agree on the accuracy and usefulness of age-adjusted PSA levels.

PSA density

This considers the relationship of the PSA level to the size of the prostate. In other words, an elevated PSA might not arouse suspicion if a man has a very enlarged prostate. The use of PSA density to interpret PSA results is controversial because cancer could possibly be overlooked in a man with an enlarged prostate.

Free versus attached PSA

PSA circulates in the blood in two forms: free, or attached to a protein molecule. With benign prostate conditions, there is more free PSA, while cancer produces more of the attached form. Researchers are exploring different ways to measure PSA and to compare these measurements in order to determine whether cancer is present.

Protein patterns

Scientists are also refining a test that can rapidly analyse the pattern of various proteins in the blood. Researchers hope that this technique can determine whether a biopsy is necessary when a person has a slightly elevated PSA level or an abnormal DRE (digital rectal examination).

OK. So research is ongoing. That's the good news. The bad news is, guess what? That's right: more tests are needed, which means further delays and even more deaths.

Zero tolerance, folks. It's a bitch! It also means, in essence, that the whole thing is back in the hands of the regulators.

Now . . . what's that big yellow thing on the wheel of my car!

8

Forum Fracas

I met Mary Harney once. I found our current Minister for Health to be warm and engaging. I also found her to be canny and wise.

It was these very qualities that people felt would help her through one of the most difficult portfolios in politics: health. It was said of her, more than once, that if anyone could get things done, it would be her.

So, it was against this backdrop that I went along to a special sitting of the Dáil, a sitting where Harney was announcing the findings of the new National Cancer Forum.

The people behind the forum had been working on a national strategy for some time and were charged with setting a blueprint for the way this dreaded disease was to be treated in Ireland in the future.

Prostate cancer must surely figure, I thought.

The Minister stood to announce the findings. Strangely, I found myself holding my breath.

Prostate screening, she informed us, and then paused, would *not* figure! In fact, the strategy would completely rule out the introduction of a population-based prostate cancer screening programme of any kind.

The words rang around the great hall with the resounding bong of a death knell. She said that the issues concerning screening had been reviewed, including the issue of prostate screening.

'The forum will advise that there is currently insufficient evidence to recommend the introduction of a population-based prostate screening programme in this country,' she said.

So, I found myself thinking, the hundreds of Irish men who die every year as a direct result of this disease are not 'evidence' enough! How many more have to die?

She went on with a concession, of sorts: the forum would advise her of emerging international evidence on prostate screening and the issue would be kept under review.

Then she set about defending the decision: 'This position [not to introduce screening] is consistent with the recommendations adopted by the European Union, which do not provide a specific recommendation for prostate screening.'

And then she got verbose: '[The EU] advocates the introduction of cancer-screening programmes which have demonstrated their efficacy with regard to professional expertise and which reflect priority-setting for health-care resources.'

I'm still trying to figure out exactly what that means. But I'm pretty sure that it wouldn't come as much consolation to the family of someone who has died as a direct result of prostate cancer.

Feel-good Factor

And then there was a strange switch in mood. The strategy was recommending that cancer services be provided around the country through four networks of hospitals. The Minister was confident that a nationwide BreastCheck service, for instance, would soon be in place.

Here was the 'feel-good' factor: the breast cancer screening programme was a 'major priority in the development of cancer services'.

The cynic would say: 'Ah, sure, those who shout loudest!' And you know what? It would certainly seem to be this way. But it *shouldn't* be this way. It's not about women and men, it's about people, and, when it comes to cancer, some people simply can't be more equal than others.

'This will ensure that all women in the relevant age group, in every county, have access to breast screening and follow-up treatment where appropriate,' the Minister continued. 'Any woman, irrespective of age or residence, who has immediate concerns or symptoms [about breast cancer] should consult her GP, who, where appropriate, will refer her to the treatment services in her area.'

So, that's it then?

No appeal? No reprieve? No hope?

Screening Strategy

Dr Liam Twomey is a different creature altogether. The former Fine Gael spokesperson on health is a big believer in screening, for all manner of ailments. On top of this, he is a doer! I've known him for a number of years, having first met him at an Association of General Practitioners Conference down in the beautiful fishing village of Carrigaline in County Cork. Carrigaline hasn't changed much down through the years. Neither has Liam Twomey. Back then, he was banging on about change. Today, he's still banging on about change.

When I approached him on the issue of prostate cancer and highlighted the fact that we don't have a screening programme for it, the doctor-turned-politician appeared to be more than a little concerned. You see, he can come at this from both angles: he has been a practising GP (a role to which he has recently returned) and knows a thing or two about the nuts and bolts of surgery life. He is also aware of the 'what happens if you catch prostate cancer too early' argument. However, he still believes that men must be given the option to make their own choices. But before that can happen, they need to be armed with all the facts.

Twomey's approach, in theory, in simple: he believes that GPs would be more than willing to fall in behind nationwide screening, provided they are properly resourced and rewarded. But acknowledging what doctors do in terms of hard cash has been a problem in this country, not just for this government, but for successive administrations.

At the end of the day, GPs have always been a little distrusted in high places because there is sometimes a tendency among politicians and civil servants to see them as business people first and physicians second.

Under the Fine Gael proposal *Future Health*, it is proposed that all adults are offered free voluntary health screening through their GP, starting from the age of twenty in the case of women and thirty in the case of men.

Tests would then be made available at five-yearly intervals until the age of fifty for women and then, subsequently, every three years until they reach the age of seventy. Similarly, men would be offered screening tests every five years until aged sixty and then every three years to the age of seventy, followed by biannual checks thereafter.

During the launch of this ambitious project, Dr Twomey outlined plans to establish a national patient database that would allow for early interventions and screening programmes on a wide range of illnesses; all of these interventions would be implemented through GP services.

There is a problem, however. 'The problem in general practice at the moment – and GPs would be the first to admit this – is that their workload and commitment is not being acknowledged,' said Dr Twomey. 'But the problems have been allowed to develop because of bad government,' he said, not being able to resist taking a little swipe.

Fine Gael leader Enda Kenny cut to the chase. He said: 'The main purpose of this new policy is that it will encourage and empower people to look after their own health.'

When it comes to prostate cancer, this would appear to be the best option we have at the moment.

Controversial Stand

The Labour Party's spokesperson on health, Liz McManus, remembers a time when people railed against the very idea of introducing a breast cancer screening programme.

'It was the exact same situation with breast-cancer prevention. People maintained that the evidence wasn't quite there and that we needed more proof that, by introducing a screening programme, we would improve the survival rate,' said McManus. 'After much kicking and screaming, the programme was eventually introduced. Prostate screening is very much in the same positon now.'

She feels, what with the alarming increase in deaths from this condition, that the Minister for Health should have stepped in to stem the tide in some way. 'She should have. But she hasn't. However, looking at things from her point of view, she is waiting on clear evidence that it will improve the lot of men before she moves on screening.'

OK. I'm a bit confused. Either the Labour Party supports screening for prostate cancer, or it doesn't. Which is it?

Liz McManus is a seasoned politician. She has been in enough scrapes to know that, when a journalist is bearing down on you, you have to leave yourself some wiggle room. There is no such thing as a black-and-white answer.

'I accept fully that screening for prostate cancer should be implemented.'

Grand.

'But it can only be implemented if we have the proof that it really works; that it really makes a difference. We're not at that point yet.'

Er, OK.

'That said, Mary Harney is certainly not doing enough on this issue. I believe it's only a matter of time before screening for prostate problems is introduced in this country. But until then, we are going to have to go through a hell of a lot of tests before it is rolled out.

'At the moment, all Mary Harney is saying is: the issue of prostate screening is controversial and, because of the controversy, we are not going to move on it.

'But just because something is controversial doesn't mean you can't explore it a little more . . . especially if it is claiming the lives of hundreds of Irish men every year.'

At the time of writing, the politicians mentioned in this chapter held their party's health portfolios.

9

House Special

On Dublin's Eccles Street – famed haunt of James Joyce – there is an organisation that the great writer would have been hard pushed to do justice to in words.

It's called ARC House, and it is a specialist cancer-support charity. For some people diagnosed with cancer, it offers a form of release; for others, it is a home away from home. Walking through the door of this magnificent Georgian building is a bit like walking back into a grander, gentler time. There is a definite atmosphere of calm about the place, due in no small measure to the people who run it.

Ursula Courtney is Director of Services at ARC House. Winner of many international awards for her work in this hugely sensitive area, and founder member of this wonderful bastion of hope for people diagnosed with the disease, Courtney has very definite views on screening for prostate cancer. And her views matter.

They matter because they are steeped in

the realities of dealing with this killer disease. They matter because she is a selfless and tireless worker for people who have lost the will to work for themselves.

Every day, she sees men, women and children who have contracted the disease. Every day, she works with them. Every day, she looks for new ways to help people play the new set of cards that life has just dealt them. Not just some days, every day.

'Should men be screened for prostate cancer? Absolutely!'

As she sits behind her desk in the magical Georgian surrounds of ARC House, there are a number of things you can't help but notice about her.

First off, she has a great face. It's one of those smiley, happy arrangements, with high cheekbones that seem to have been designed to support a perpetual smile. It's the kind of face that just makes you want to smile right back.

The other thing you notice is her attitude. It's one of those all-too-rare 'can do' attitudes. It comes off her in great, palpable waves. Courtney doesn't deal in 'pie in the sky'. She is grounded, pragmatic and practical. But equally, she represents a little pool of hope in what can be a raging river of despair.

'The thing about prostate screening,' she says, pulling herself up in her seat and pushing in a little closer to me, 'is that it is extremely cost-effective. I mean, what are we talking about here? We're talking about a simple blood test, for God's sake! It's something that any GP could do, with the minimum of fuss. I'm sure that there are many GPs doing it already, but not in an orchestrated way. And this is part of the problem.'

She does feel, however, that if the issue could be sorted by a simple blood test, we would be home and dry on prostate screening. The big problem, she feels, centres mainly on the issue of the dreaded digital rectal exam (DRE).

'Let's call a spade a spade,' she says, the pragmatic Ursula beginning to emerge. 'People are going to make the comparison with breast screening for women and prostate screening for men. But it's not the same. Women are used to having their breasts touched or examined. But men are not used to anybody going anywhere near that area,' she says, nodding vigorously in the direction of my nether-regions. 'If it weren't for DRE, I think a lot more men would be presenting to have their prostate checked out.'

It's a point well made. Some time ago, the *Pulse* Health Squad were over in the west of the country making a documentary on men's health for RTÉ TV. We had just finished filming, when the GP in whose surgery we were shooting began to talk about the potential dangers of ignoring signs of prostate 'abnormalities'. At which point he turned to the camera crew. The two unfortunates just happened to be in an 'at risk' group: they were both aged circa forty-five.

'Tell you what,' says the GP to the guy holding the camera, 'hop up on the couch and I'll do a quick DRE, just to be on the safe side.'

The cameraman's face drained of all natural colour and turned a paler shade of white. A paler shade of white is not a good colour.

'What! Me?' he spluttered in protest. 'When you say "DRE", doc, I assume you mean the finger-up-the-bum job?'

'I do,' said our intrepid physician, already beginning to pull on the rubber glove. The snap of the rubber reverberated around the suddenly silent room like the crack of a whip.

'Let me put it to you this way, doctor,' said our camera guy, emphasising the word 'doctor' for effect and falling over chairs as he backed awkwardly out of the room, 'if you come near me with that finger, say goodbye to the finger!'

Courtney laughs at the story. But she's not surprised.

'Typical! Men have a problem when it comes to this kind of examination. But the thing we have to stress is that it is *not* painful. At most, it might be a little uncomfortable, but there is no pain associated with it. We need to let people know this. We need to raise awareness.'

Poor Visitors

When it comes to men's health, the prostate is a small part of a much bigger picture. Men are notoriously poor visitors to their GP surgery. In fact, a lot of health-related articles are now being 'placed' in women's magazines, because health watchdogs feel that the best way to get a man to a GP surgery is to get his wife or partner to drag him along!

'Why are men bad at going to the doctor? Because of fear,' says Courtney. 'It's the old head-in-the-sand attitude. Simply put, they just feel that if they ignore the problem, it will go away. There can also be a huge element of denial in the whole process.'

Courtney, who runs special men's-heath group sessions in ARC House, feels that men as a rule don't really like to talk about health-related issues. 'It can be seen as weak, particularly if the conversation begins to drift anywhere south of the waist.'

Small Shadow

Psychiatrist David Leahy has issues with the whole principle of DRE. A thoughtful, gentle man, he likes to sit back for a time and think about his answers. A small shadow crosses his face at the notion of the examination.

'Why do most men baulk at the very idea of a finger up the rectum? Because it's an extremely invasive thing. More than this, it can also be very humiliating. In a sense, you are required to be very submissive. A lot of men are not good with submission; it goes against the grain.'

Putting on his psychiatrist's hat, he explores the connotations. 'Think about it: you are required to lie in the foetal position, with your legs drawn up underneath you. The person doing the examination is behind you, in what could be termed a position of power.'

Cork physician Dr Robert Gaffney feels that there are two main issues surrounding DRE. 'Most men like to feel that they are their own person, that they own their body, and they don't want anything shoved inside it. They can't deal with this sort of invasion.'

He also feels that many men have this in-built 'violation' valve hot-wired into the circuitry of their brain. 'I think that there is a definite homophobic thing going on with a lot of these men. Not only do they project this, they would rather go without the procedure – and its inherent health benefits – than face up to the prospect of DRE.'

OK. Let's put it to the ultimate test . . .

10

A Testing Time

I'm in the Beacon Clinic, a private health facility on Dublin's south side that specialises in routine health checks. The atmosphere is friendly and comforting.

There are a couple of men sitting in the waiting area with me. They are well dressed and flicking through copies of business magazines.

I have decided, seeing as I am conducting an investigation into the benefits of prostate screening, that, really, I should get myself checked out. Practice first, preach later.

I get the old once-over (heart, lung function, reflexes, and so on), and then I steer the doctor towards my interest in the prostate.

'Well,' he says, 'we'll have to check your PSA levels first and then we'll have a stab at the DRE.'

He giggles every so slightly at his 'stab' joke. I'm not laughing.

And I'm not alone. Most men wouldn't

even countenance the idea of being 'penetrated' in any way, shape or form. Keep your finger to yourself! I want to scream. But I know that the DRE (digital rectal exam) is an essential part of a proper prostate investigation.

There are two approaches that doctors think of immediately when examining the prostate. The first is the Prostate Specific Antigen test. The second is DRE. Because the prostate is situated close to the rectum, the best way in is . . . through the rectum!

OK. I admit that even the prospect of it is not the most enticing. I'd rather be fishing, and I don't fish. In fact, I'd rather be doing just about anything else. But, needs must. I decide to lie back and think of England.

The snap of the rubber glove signifies that you have crossed the line. There is no way back; he's going in!

One word of advice at this point . . . *relax*! The more uptight you are, the more difficult it is going to be for the doctor to learn what he needs to learn. Essentially, what he is feeling for are little lumps and bumps on the prostate itself. As Billy Connolly puts it: 'He's trying to determine whether or not your prostate has turned from a bagel into a donut.'

This is a useful analogy for the way in which an unhealthy prostate changes shape. But if there are irregular protrusions, this will not tell the full story.

A DRE is a useful tool in the doctor's armoury. But it is far from perfect, because some small cancers (hiding away in corners) can be missed, as it's only the bottom and the sides of the prostate that can be examined in this way.

'So, how are you doing there,' asks the doctor, moving into position.

'Honestly,' I say, 'I have been better.'

'There's nothing to it. You'll see,' he says, sensing my feeling of impending doom.

As the finger goes in, the sensation is one of pressure, not pain. The more you relax, the easier it becomes. I stop thinking of England and start working with him.

'So,' I say, warming strangely to the situation, 'found anything untoward yet? I lost a watch a few weeks back.'

Suddenly the finger is out and, honestly, I feel no trauma, either physical or emotional. Yes, folks, I can safely say that there will be no mental scarring. And it has to be said that I do feel a bit easier that, for the moment, I don't appear to have any doughnuts up my butt!

He takes the glove off and informs me, gleefully, that everything seems fine, and then he loses himself in the PSA reading that has jut landed on his desk.

Simply put, a PSA is a blood test that is designed to look for a protein that the prostate makes. As a matter of course, a healthy prostate makes a little bit of

PSA. A prostate that is being attacked by cancer makes a little bit more. As the cancer gets worse, more PSA is made. In this way, a doctor can chart the course and severity of the cancer.

The PSA test is not perfect on its own, however. There are certain forms of tumour that grow on, and in, the prostate that won't elevate PSA levels. And there are some other processes, like benign prostatic hyperplasia, that can cause the PSA to be falsely elevated, without any cancer being present. One thing is true, nonetheless: the higher your PSA reading, the more likely you are to have prostate cancer.

OK, let's pull all these strands together. If your PSA level is elevated, you may or may not have prostate cancer. If your DRE is 'suspicious', you may or may not have cancer. If both your PSA is elevated and your DRE is 'suspicious', you will definitely need further investigation. There is really only one way to know for sure if you have prostate cancer, and that is to have a biopsy taken and sent for analysis.

Let's look a little closer at the PSA reading. The cut-off point for most doctors is a reading of 4.0 ng/ml. This means that anything below that is normal and anything above it is abnormal.

Professor Fred Stephens puts it in even simpler terms: 'PSA levels in blood are measured in "units" of one microgram per litre. This has been found to be a very convenient measurement. The normal upper limit of PSA in men up to about the age of fifty is 2.5. By the time you reach sixty years of age, a reading of 3.5 might be considered normal. By the time you reach eighty years old, a reading of 10 could be considered normal.' This is because, as you get older, the size of the prostate is increasing exponentially.

My reading is at the lower end of low; so, for the moment, I'm not a cause for concern. However, my doctor persists with the investigation by delving into signs and symptoms. And the little tell-tale pointers that there could be something amiss are easy enough to read. They include:

§ trouble getting urine to flow;

§ urinating more frequently than usual;

§ the feeling that you can't empty all of your bladder, no matter how hard you try;

§ pain on urination, or on ejaculation;

§ blood in your urine or semen;

§ impotence;

§ bone pain.

Professor Stephens frames the importance of acting on the symptoms. 'The earlier a patient seeks medical attention for anything unusual or different, the more likely it will be that any cancer will be detected at a curable stage,' he says.

An obstruction in the normal flow of urine is one of the most telling factors, it could be argued. Professor Stephens says that the flow may be slow to start and slow to stop, and that there may also be incontinence. He says that, added to this, there can be an urge to pass urine several times a night. Occasionally, there may be a complete obstruction because the enlarged prostate is pressing on the urethra.

Prostate cancer, like any other cancer, can spread. The most common site of spread and secondary growth of this cancer is the bone. Bone pain associated with prostate cancer can be incredibly painful. The bones most commonly affected are the vertebrae in the back, the bones in the pelvis and the large thigh bone (the femur). Having said that, any bone in the body can be targeted.

Doctors are great folks for categorising and dividing things up into stages. They have done the same with prostate cancer. In fact, prostate cancer is divided into four different stages, in a bid to help guide treatments and offer appropriate information about cure chances.

Stage I

The tumour cannot be felt during a Digital Rectal Examination. It can only be detected by an elevated PSA blood test, or stumbled upon during another prostate procedure for a benign (harmless) condition.

Stage II

The tumour can be felt during a DRE, but it has not spread beyond the prostate itself.

Stage III

The tumour has extended outside the prostate and can be in the seminal vesicles, but not in any other organs or lymph nodes.

Stage IV

The tumour has spread to other organs or lymph nodes.

If your stage, grade, or PSA is high enough, you may be referred for other tests before treatment.

Tests like CT scans can examine the prostate and localised lymph nodes. Some patients are referred for a bone scan, which uses a radioactive tracer to look for metastasis (spread) to any of the bones.

If a doctor is very worried about the possible spread to lymph nodes, you may be asked to undergo a surgical lymph-node sampling before proceeding with any definitive treatment.

One of the big criticisms levelled at men is the fact that they don't like going to the doctor in the first place. There are a number of reasons for this reticence. One is that they feel they don't really know what to ask.

Well, just to knock this particular excuse on the head, here are a number of questions you can ask your GP when you go for that all-important prostate exam:

§ Could my symptoms be a sign of cancer?

§ What tests do you recommend?

§ Why?

§ If I don't have cancer, what can I do to alleviate these symptoms?

§ If I do have cancer, what stage is it at?

§ What is my PSA level?

§ Would it be useful to get a second opinion?

§ What is my prognosis?

§ Is it likely to recur?

§ Do I need additional tests to look for lymph-node involvement or metastases?

§ What are my treatment options?

§ What are the possible side effects?

§ How can these side effects be managed?

§ Are there clinical trials that would be appropriate for me?

§ What other specialists should I talk to?

11

This Is Cancer!

Prostate cancer is no different from any other cancer. It takes hold. Then it spreads, bullying surrounding tissues and organs to give up their vital space. True, by and large, prostate cancer spreads more slowly than most other cancers; but, nonetheless, it follows the same general pattern as that of any other form of malignancy.

So, if we are to understand the whys and wherefores of prostate cancer, we first have to get back to basics and ask one fundamental question: what is cancer?

The medical dictionaries are quite black and white about it. They tell us that cancers arise from the abnormal and uncontrolled division of cells, which then go on to invade and destroy the surrounding tissues. But this is not cancer.

They tell us that there are many causative factors, including tobacco, which is associated with lung cancer;

76

radiation, which is linked to some forms of bone cancers and leukaemia. There are also several viruses that are known to cause tumours. But this is not cancer.

They tell us that there may be a genetic element in the development of cancer. They point out that in more than half of all cancers, a gene identified by the number 'p57' is deleted or impaired. The normal function of this gene is to prevent the uncontrolled division of cells. But this is not cancer.

Some dictionaries will even point to a condition known as cancer phobia – a personality disorder that leads to compulsively performed rituals, like avoiding air that has already been breathed by others, or the avoidance of people in general. Cancer phobia can result in the sufferer turning minor symptoms into major malignancies, accompanied by severe panic attacks. But this is not cancer.

Cancer is a disease that often takes over the heart and the mind of those unfortunate enough to be diagnosed with the condition. Cancer takes up residence in tormented emotions. Cancer is in the face of its victims. That's what cancer is really all about. Cancer is hell!

Home from Home

I went back to Dublin's Eccles Street to visit ARC House again and meet some of the people there. After my general tour, I got talking to one young woman who was sitting in the drawing room looking out onto the manicured gardens. I remember that she had a porcelain face and a slight frame. She had been diagnosed with cancer of the colon just a few months prior to our conversation. She was nineteen.

She asked all the usual questions; experienced all the usual physical and emotional pain; screamed at God; and pulled her hair out before the chemotherapy could perform that particular indignity for her.

She had been a student in Trinity College, but the disease (and the rigours of the treatment) ate into her energy supplies, and she had to resign from the course. If nothing else, this gave her time to think.

'Cancer is something that I have,' she said, locking onto me with a look that said: I'm still here fighting. 'It's not me. I don't define myself by it. But I can't get away from the fact that it is there.'

She was a fighter all right. Determination was etched into her tiny features like a badge of honour. She was saying all the right things. But there was also a palpable sadness about her. She appeared trapped by it, straitjacketed by it, because, no matter how many times she asked the question 'Why me?', the answer could never do justice to the inexorable, creeping, horrible reality.

The physical pain that people go

through when they hear a diagnosis of cancer is almost always not only matched but surpassed by the emotional torment.

According to leading cancer counsellor Joel Nathan, there are a number of reactions that can follow a diagnosis. He says we can feel trapped, numb, guilty, confused, sad, lonely, anxious, panicky and scared. The list, it would appear, goes on and on.

'Abruptly confronted by the fear of our own death and the manner of our dying, we can be cut off from those we love and the things with which we are familiar,' says Nathan. 'In a flash, our dreams and plans for the future are torn from our grasp and, like sailors in a storm, we find ourselves adrift without oars, without a compass, and unaware where the tide will take us. The despair can be unimaginable.'

Nathan captures the emotional desert of a diagnosis of cancer perfectly in his brilliant book *What To Do When They Say It's Cancer* (mentioned above). He points out that you can't will away your responses and feelings, and that it is essential to your eventual recovery (because people *do* recover) that you recognise these responses as normal.

'You also need to give expression to your moods and feelings rather than bottling them up, so they do not overwhelm you. This is important, because unexpressed emotions drain you of energy and keep you focused on controlling them instead of directing your resources towards your recovery.'

He says the only way through is to 'honour your feelings' and remind yourself that they will pass. 'Be gentle on yourself,' he writes, 'even if you feel that you can't keep two simple thoughts together.'

Strange Thing

Outside in the ARC House gardens, a little woman is digging at the ground with a hoe. She is dressed in a waist-length denim jacket and a pair of jeans. The ensemble is finished off with a pair of green wellies. She gently scrapes the earth into place and paws it into a mound with her bare hands.

She sees me coming towards her, and stops. 'Hello,' she says, an enormous smile lighting up her face, like sun suddenly peering out from behind a cloud. Her teeth are brilliant white, but her face is parched and a little cracked, like a plot of ground that has been exposed to the elements for too long. Although we haven't been introduced, she seems to know who I am and why I am there.

She walks over to the corner of the garden, where bunches of baby flowers are gathered together in a riot of colour, bobbing madly in the breeze. She grabs a handful and walks back towards me. 'You know,' she says, bending down to plant the flowers in the freshly made bed, 'cancer is a strange thing.'

I don't know who this woman is. Somehow it doesn't seem to matter who she is, I find I just want to listen to what she has to say. She seems very much at ease with herself. Strangely, I begin to feel at ease as well. Her voice has a melodic English reverb to it. She stands up again and looks up at the sky.

'Living with fear is like having a dark cloud hanging over your life and your mind. It shuts out everything. It blots out dreams. It can smother hope. But in time, the fear subsides and other feelings take its place. And that's OK, because you really have to go with whatever you are feeling.'

She is back down on the ground again, patting at the earth, pulling the flowers into place. 'Yeah,' she says, 'cancer is strange. It's like being suddenly set adrift on a choppy sea. You look around but can't see anybody, because the waves are so big and so strong. You feel as though you are going to go under; but you bob back up again. People are so resilient.'

She pauses for a time and cups the flowers to her face, breathing deeply. 'I think it is important to continue on with your life as normally as you can. Sure, you're going to be battered by the harsh winds of terror and uncertainty. Sometimes it's hard to think about anything other than the cancer; but you will feel better if you just keep going. I know I did.'

She gets back up to her feet and arches the small of her back to iron out the creaks. She starts to walk back to the corner to get more flowers, and then stops and turns towards me again. 'There is one other thing. Learn to laugh. Laughter can be very helpful. It can be life-enhancing. It can give you a sense of survival rather than despair.'

And there's that brilliant smile again.

12

The Phone Call

It hadn't been a good day, and it was about to get a whole lot worse.

I had just come from a specially convened cancer conference in Dublin Castle, an austere structure with hard cobbled stones and an even harder history. In keeping with the theme, the conference had some hard news for the pro-screening contingent.

The British government's 'Cancer Tsar', Professor Michael Richards, was in attendance. Richards, as well as being one of the leading cancer commentators in the world, sports the kind of looks that would drive some Hollywood actors wild with jealousy. When he walks into a room, people can't help but look at him.

Turns out that the man would rather throw his weight behind a bowel cancer screening programme than a prostate programme.

Why? Well, the evidence for prostate

screening is a little thin on the ground, he says.

'There is no [randomised controlled] test that shows screening would save lives,' he says. 'In fact, there is a real risk that it could do as much harm as good.'

Oh? How so?

'Because it will undoubtedly find cancers, but those cancers might very well not have caused a problem during the patient's lifetime.'

So we're back to the old 'watchful waiting' scenario. In fairness, the good professor is also concerned about the fallout from invasive anti-prostate procedures, which can include impotence and incontinence.

He is pro-choice: preferring to let the patient choose for himself which way to proceed. 'My position is that we should provide information about PSA tests and let men make their own informed decisions.'

On bowel-cancer screening he is a lot clearer: 'For bowel cancer, there are now four trials, all of which effectively show the same thing: you can reduce the death rate in the affected population by about 15 percent through screening.'

He said that people will argue about which type of screening to introduce. However, the important thing is that they do not go on arguing, but that they get to it. This is exactly what I want him to say about prostate screening. But he stops short.

After the meeting, a woman approaches me. She has the kind of smile that would light up the room if the electricity failed. Strangely, it seems out of place in this gathering.

She moves conspiratorially close, and says: 'You do know that the whole issue of prostate screening is not about moral right or wrong; it's about resources.'

'Really?' I say, stepping back from her just a little so that I can buy myself some space. 'What do you mean exactly by "resources"?'

'You know,' she says, moving in close again, 'urologists, technology, extra clinical staff, extra admin staff, marketing . . . .'

She stops for a beat, trying to gauge my reaction, and then continues. 'You do know that prostate cancer is so far down the list of Department of Health priorities that it doesn't really register.'

Not far short of a thousand men will die in Ireland this year because of this disease . . . and it doesn't even register with the people who can do something about it! Jeeze!

'Sorry,' I say, 'but I never got your name. Who are you?'

'Oh,' she says, flashing me the dazzling smile once more and beginning to walk off. 'Nobody.'

Suddenly, I feel a bit drained.

The Consequences

Outside, the darkness of the evening has descended, and the little inner-city streets are choked with traffic. As I walk to my train, the professor's words are running over and over in my head.

He says he is all for choice when it comes to men making decisions about prostate treatment. He also says that screening for prostate cancer will, undoubtedly, reveal some malignancies. He is worried, justifiably, about the consequences of going in after cancer growing in the prostate – and setting off things like incontinence and impotence.

So, here's the choice: incontinence and impotence, or a painful death. If I had prostate cancer, I would like to be in a position to make that choice. So, I imagine, would John B. Keane.

But first, I would have to know if I had prostate cancer or not . . . which brings us right back to screening.

The professor said that 'tests show that screening for bowel cancer can save lives'. Tests show! The tests are the key, then.

I put in a quick call to the Irish Cancer Society to find out if there are any prostate-screening tests planned for Ireland. I'm told that they'll get back to me.

Rattling Cages

To screen, or not to screen? My head was still mulling over the ramifications when my mobile phone rang.

'Is that Rory Hafford?'

'Yes it is. Who is this?'

'Never mind who this is. Just listen.'

I'm usually good with voices. This one I couldn't place. It was educated, like a doctor's voice (and I've dealt with enough of them). It was forthright, to the point, and with a distinctly sinister edge.

'You've been asking a lot of questions about prostate screening, and you've been rattling quite a few cages.'

'Hold on. Rattling cages? I'm just trying to find out if it would be feasible to introduce a screening programme to Ireland,' I said, trying to stay calm, trying to get the image out of my head that I had somehow wandered onto the set of a gangster movie!

'Your problem is that you like the sound of your own voice too much. Just shut up and listen for a change . . . it could save you a lot of trouble . . . '

'Trouble? What kind of trouble?'

'I'll tell you what kind of trouble. Firstly, you don't know what you're talking about. Secondly, the infrastructure does not exist in this country to support a screening programme of this magnitude. Furthermore, there are more pressing matters than prostate cancer . . . '

'Hold on a minute,' I said, 'there are more pressing problems than hundreds of Irish men dying of a disease that they could have done something about had they known they had the disease in the first place?'

'There you go again, blabbing your mouth off without first engaging your brain. I'm just going to give you two words of advice: back off!'

Click. The phone went dead. A strange, surreal feeling washed over me. I felt like I was being watched. I looked around, suddenly terrified. Nothing stood out. Just the usual collection of souls plugged into their iPods, rustling the pages of worn novels and shuffling from one foot to the other, bored with waiting for the train to arrive.

At that point, I thought seriously about walking away from the whole thing. It would be the wise thing to do. It would definitely be the safest thing to do. You don't mess with medical muscle.

And then my phone rang again.

'Hello.'

'Oh, hi. Is that Rory Hafford?'

Jesus, I thought, here we go again.

'Yes,' I said, tentatively.

'It's John Armstrong from the Cancer Society. I believe you were looking for me.'

13

Laughing Matters

So here's Bob Monkhouse sitting on the *Parkinson* show, making light of his brush with prostate cancer.

'I went to my doctor and he said: "The news is not good . . . you have ten to live." 'Ten?' I said. 'What do you mean, ten? Ten what? Ten weeks? Ten months?'

'The doctor looks at his watch and says: "Ten, nine, eight, seven . . . "'

Funny man; funny routine. And humour is as good a way as any of getting a very serious message across.

Monkhouse is not the only comic to broach the subject through laughter. The great Billy Connolly is another who has gone to his GP and tried to see the funny side of the prostate check-up.

His stage routine goes something like this: 'So, I went to my doctor to have my prostate checked out. You know, the old finger up the bum, or, as it is known, the "urologist's handshake".

'When he inserted his finger, I thought: "Oh my God, he's found a dead tree and shoved it up my arse!"'

(Connolly puts his finger, as it were, on a very real problem: the fear and loathing most men have of someone inserting a finger up their back passage – even for health reasons!)

The two sketches were played as an introduction to a recent media-awareness campaign on the prostate. The campaign was organised by the British Prostate Cancer Charity (PCC) and rolled out in the UK.

Across the water, the main problem the British have with prostate cancer can be summed up in one word: ignorance!

For openers, there is ignorance among the male population there, which has not yet come to terms with talking openly about intimate issues.

There is also ignorance in the education system: an alarming 10 percent of Britons are under the impression that women also have a prostate!

Then there is ignorance and disagreement among the medical establishment in the UK, which has not yet agreed on the best way to diagnose and treat prostate-cancer patients.

Writing in the *Guardian* newspaper, prostate-cancer sufferer and PCC worker Phil Baldy tries to put the problem into perspective: 'Women take care of their bodies in a way that men just don't. Before my diagnosis, I had a basic idea of

anatomy, but I'd have had a problem pointing to my prostate gland on a drawing.'

Phil Baldy is not alone. With about
10,000 men dying in the UK every year from
this disease (that's about one death every
hour), prostate cancer is the second-
biggest killer of men in that country,
topped only by lung cancer.

Yet, according to the PCC, 90 percent
of adults in the UK don't have a clue what
the prostate gland actually does, or where
you would find it.

Baldy feels that part of the problem
lies in the fact that the prostate has a
sexual function (in that it produces some
of the fluid that makes up semen). 'Men
like to think of themselves as super-
studs,' says Baldy. 'Anything that goes
wrong below the belt, they just ignore.'

Another problem, according to the PCC,
is the way prostate cancer is treated in
the UK. Prostate patients are more dissat-
isfied with their medical treatment than
those suffering from any other ailment and
are almost twice as likely as other
patients not to be informed about the side
effects of their treatments, even though
these can cause long-term problems like
impotence and incontinence.

Yet there are many ways to treat
prostate problems (around ten, at the last
count). Two of the main ones are
brachytherapy, which involves the inser-
tion of tiny radioactive-iodine seeds
into the prostate itself. These seeds give

off cancer-killing radiation in little pulses. Another method of treating the problem is using cryotherapy, a process designed to freeze and then thaw the prostate rapidly, breaking the cancer cells apart.

Irish Pulling Power

Irish radio personality Gerry Ryan gets himself into some awkward situations, almost on a daily basis. All you have to do is tune into his hit programme on any given day, and you'll find the man talking about all manner of 'taboo' subjects, in a way that suggests that, really, he couldn't give a toss what people think of him. The more outrageous, the better. It's just one of the reasons why his show is top of the pile.

With pulling power like this, people like Gerry Ryan are a hugely valuable asset when it comes to getting an important message across to the public. With this in mind, perhaps, Gerry rowed in behind the recent Irish public-awareness campaign on prostate cancer. It's a subject that the man has a lot of time for.

Gerry dealt with the subject at some length on his morning programme and posed for pictures with leading Irish urological surgeon Dr Thomas Lynch. When it comes to prostate awareness, Dr Lynch likes to cut to the chase.

'We need more urologists to deal with

this condition. It's as simple as that,' he says. 'With the number of urologists on or about twenty-three at the moment [figures correct at the time of writing], we have only half the required number of these specialists in Ireland. Over the next number of years, when men's health takes on a higher profile, hopefully the number of urologists will be increased.'

The awareness campaign highlighted some worrying statistics: the number of men being diagnosed every year with prostate cancer has nearly doubled since the mid-1990s – and doctors are now demanding that a special 'medical investigation' be carried out to find out why.

The figures are stark: there were around 1,000 new prostate cancers annually back in 1994. But in recent years, this figure has climbed to 1,800. The incidence of this killer of men is increasing by about 6 percent every year.

Dr Harry Comber, Director of the National Cancer Registry, doesn't feel that this major hike in figures could be described as a 'natural increase'. In fact, he believes that we are finding more prostate cancers because more men are presenting for PSA testing. This fact aside, however, he is still not convinced that screening is the way to go in Ireland.

Speaking in the *Irish Times*, he said: 'There is no consensus on a national PSA screening programme [in Ireland]. Evidence suggests that, for this type of cancer, picking it up earlier may not make a big difference to the patient. It may be an issue that resources should not be directed at it because it is not benefiting anybody.'

Dr Comber says that the focus of research has shifted slightly to the north of the country because, unlike the rest of Ireland, the north has not experienced an upsurge in prostate-cancer rates. An investigation to determine why this is the case will examine the number of men presenting themselves for testing, how those diagnosed with the disease are followed up, and the outcome of treatment. This study will take 'a number of years', according to Dr Comber.

Worryingly, the increase in prostate-cancer figures is mirrored right across the cancer spectrum in Ireland. The report *Cancer in Ireland 1994-2001* shows that the number of cancer cases is increasing by 2.3 percent a year, from 19,290 in 1994 to 22,473 in 2001. There were an average of 20,523 cases of cancer reported every year over that period.

Because of the lack of a screening programme in this country, the onus is on men to go and get themselves checked out. But Dr Thomas Lynch feels that this is resulting in many men 'sticking their head in the sand and doing nothing about it'.

'It is very sad when I meet a man of sixty with an advanced stage of the disease who could have been diagnosed five or six years earlier and could have had it cured by an operation,' says Dr Lynch. 'Prostate cancer is, if caught at an early stage, potentially curable. Just like breast cancer in women.'

He stops just short of advocating a screening programme for Ireland. 'I'm not saying it won't be worth our while in a few years' time. There are ongoing studies in centres in the UK into this issue. And because the population in England and Ireland is so similar, whatever we learn from England we can extrapolate and apply to this country.'

The good news, with the Irish awareness campaign, is that most of the newspapers and electronic media outlets picked up on the story. The danger is that the message will simply come . . . and go. There needs to be constant vigilance on this issue.

As part of the campaign, AstraZeneca, one of the more progressive pharmaceutical companies, took the opportunity to launch a new leaflet on the subject. And they adopted an approach that is close to the heart of most men: a motors theme!

AstraZeneca asked one pertinent question: Do you know what goes on under your bonnet?

'As we get older, our bodies may not appear to be the very latest in driving technology. But even an older model can still run like a dream, if properly maintained,' went the AstraZeneca message. 'That's why it's important that the more

circuits we have completed, the more frequently we go in for a service. Only then
can we be sure that our prostate stays in
good working order.'

The AstraZeneca campaign highlighted
the, at times, subtle difference between
a benign enlarged prostate (BPH) and
prostate cancer. 'The trouble is that men
with early prostate cancer are unlikely to
have symptoms and must be prostate-aware.
When symptoms do occur, they are very similar to those of BPH. They may be the
signs of prostate cancer and, therefore,
if you have noticed any of the ftell-tale
signs (see page 169), you should pull into
the pits immediately for an inspection.'

14

The Choice

The Irish Cancer Society is the first port of call for many people worried about the disease. The society's headquarters, nestling among the leafy tree-lined streets just off Dublin's Northumberland Road, was set up as an information-giver and a supporter of people with cancer. Prostate cancer, however, does not seem to be at the top of their agenda.

In fact, their approach to the condition is summed up – officially – in just two sentences. For the record, here are those two sentences: 'The Irish Cancer Society's view on prostate-cancer screening is that men who are over the age of fifty (especially those who have a positive family history of prostate cancer) and are concerned should consult with their GP about the merits of screening. Screening involves a physical examination and blood test, which measures the PSA (Prostate Specific Antigen).'

Essentially, what the society is saying in this case is that, if men are worried about prostate cancer, they should get up off their behind and make all the running themselves. They should then 'consult with their GP about the merits of screening'.

This begs the question: to what end? GPs don't know anything about the merits of screening for prostate cancer in this country, because nobody has bothered to do any Irish studies.

I'm not happy with the society. I decide to get a little bolshy with them. But they cut me off mid-rant: if I need more information on the society's position with regard to prostate screening, I should contact Professor John Armstrong in St Luke's Hospital.

Now I feel a little easier. I remember John Armstrong from a few years back: a focused sort of an individual, and certainly the kind of medic who would instil confidence in his patients.

That's the good news. The not-so-good news is that I also seem to remember him being very evidence-based. For that reason alone, I can't see him advocating screening.

I couldn't have been more wrong!

John Armstrong has the kind of face that belongs on someone a lot younger! When you are introduced to him as 'Professor', you think: 'Yeah, right!' He looks, for all the world, like he is just out of medical school, and you're left scratching your head as to how he managed to cram in a professorship on top of everything else, and in such a short space of time.

Nonetheless, *Professor* John Armstrong it is, specialist in radiation oncology at my old alma mater, University College Dublin.

When I raise the issue of screening with him, he suddenly becomes bullish. It's as though, instinctively, he knows where I'm coming from and is determined to get there ahead of me.

'"Why don't we have screening?" is too simple a question,' he says, fixing me with a hard stare. 'You have to ask yourself what kind of people are now the opinion-makers in Irish medicine. I'll tell you what kind of people: they are the same people I went to medical school with. They are steeped in the philosophy of "hold what you have". They went to college at a time when money, and budgets, were everything.'

He stops for a beat to check that I am still with him. He is animated. A fire burns behind his eyes. He continues. 'When they came out of medical school and into their first job, they were actually rewarded with a bonus if they didn't spend their budgets. That thinking is, to a large degree, still prevalent today – and it is part of the reason why we don't have a screening programme for prostate cancer.'

He says that running in tandem with the 'let's hold what we have' approach is a worrying 'let's do nothing' approach. As he says it, the dreadful term 'watchful waiting' looms large in my mind.

'For a country with such great ties to America, we couldn't be further from their thinking when it comes to the medical management of some conditions, prostate cancer being a prime example. The Americans have the exact opposite of our 'do nothing' approach; they want to do everything they can to offset long-term complications. They attack this problem head-on.

'In Ireland, sadly, we have an in-built resistance to proactive medicine. In relation to prostate screening, there is a resistance to creating the infrastructure to deal with the problem; there is a resistance to invasive treatment options; there is a resistance to funding even a pilot screening programme.

'Would it be a good thing if we actively took all these steps? Absolutely, it would. But they don't want it to be a good thing. They want things to stay as they are. They want the status quo.'

Gathering Momentum

The professor's point is well made. According to the latest dispatch from the UCI Medical Center in California, the move towards mandatory prostate screening is gathering considerable momentum.

'PROSTATE SCREENING COULD SAVE YOUR LIFE' screams the headline from the very latest UCI medical bulletin.

'At the early stages [of prostate cancer], it's 90-95 percent curable,' says Dr Allen Shanbreg, Professor of Surgery and Urology at UCI Medical Center and a renowned expert in the diagnosis and treatment of the condition. 'It's in the later stages that the survival/cure rate goes down dramatically.'

Thanks to special research approaches like those at UCI Medical, screening programmes that detect early stages of prostate cancer are significantly better today than in the past. The proof is that of the approximately 300,000 American men diagnosed with prostate cancer this year, 85 percent will survive.

Dr Thomas Ahlering, a urologic oncologist at UCI Medical Center, says that because the incidence of prostate cancer increases as we get older, he believes firmly that it would be a good idea if annual PSA blood-test screenings are made mandatory for men over the age of fifty – and for men over forty who have risk factors like a family history of the disease.

It may also be important to note that because of the wide range of treatment options – ranging from laparoscopic lymph node dissection to radiation and cryosurgery – the UCI Medical Center is an important address to have in your book if you or someone close to you is diagnosed with prostate cancer.

The UCI bulletin says that while doctors may approach the issue of prostate cancer from different directions, they all seem to agree on one thing: 'Early detection opens the door to more treatment options and a far greater chance of survival.'

Prostate cancer is the number-two killer of men in the US after lung cancer. It affects 190,000 men and kills almost 30,000 each and every year. However, death rates have been falling each year for the last five years – a decline some doctors attribute to PSA testing.

The UCI Medical Center's slogan is 'A Passion for Care'. Maybe it's this that makes all the difference.

Closer to home, a study published recently in the *British Medical Journal* followed the fortunes of fifty-two men in the UK who underwent the PSA test. Of that number, forty-eight said that they would encourage other men to go through the same process.

The men said that they weren't that concerned about the lack of absolute evidence that prostate screening could save their life. They were more concerned that by having the test done, they were acting responsibly, they were accessing the latest health information in relation to

their prostate, and they were avoiding
possible regrets about not taking the
test.

My heart is singing. Here is one of the
most influential oncologists in the country saying out loud what every right-
thinking medic in Ireland must surely be
thinking. I decide to tie him down even
further. I repeat my mantra: 'So, John,
let me just get this straight. You agree
that if you look for something, you have
a better chance of finding it? You agree
that prostate cancer is like any other
cancer in that if you find it early and
go in after it, you have a better chance
of an effective outcome? You agree that,
in principle, we should have a screening
programme in Ireland?'

He fixes me with that familiar hard
stare of his. 'Look,' he says, 'everything
you say is correct. In fact, there is not
a shred of evidence against it.'

He illustrates his point with an example. 'Take the issue of cervical cancer.
There is a massive push to raise awareness
of this condition and to roll out screening programmes for women. Why should cervical cancer be any different from
prostate cancer?

'It is not my intention to set male
against female. Good luck to women and all
their health endeavours; I would be the
first to applaud them. However, why should
men be any different? This is not a gender thing, this is a health thing. Men,

women: we are all equal citizens and everyone should be given equal treatment.'

He has seen this kind of thing before. 'This is classic Irish foot-dragging. Even if we kicked off now with some pilot projects, it would be ten to fifteen years before a viable screening programme would be in place.'

He stops. Gets up. Walks around for a bit. Looks out the window. His mind is going at a fair clip. You can see it. He turns to me again. 'As far as I can see, the choice is simple: a modest financial outlay to carry out a number of Irish pilot projects, or the death of hundreds of Irish men every year. That's the choice.'

Since this chapter was written, the Irish Cancer Society has become more active on the issue of prostate cancer, helped in no small measure by the likes of journalists George Hook and Gerry Ryan. The society now runs regular awareness initiatives, but stops short of calling for screening.

15

Our Own National Screening

Centre . . . Ready to Go!

Dr Herb Joiner-Bey is an outspoken American doctor who is horrified at the manner in which prostate cancer is treated in Ireland. On a whistle-stop tour of the 'Emerald Isle' to promote his research into the medical use of flax oil, he was alarmed to hear that there was no screening pro-gramme in place here to catch the disease at a stage at which something concrete could be done to treat it effectively.

'That's shocking! In the States, the approach is all towards being proactive in conditions like prostate cancer,' Joiner-Bey told me. 'I think it is very remiss if you don't offer people a way of detecting that they might just be in the grip of a disease that could actually kill them.'

He speaks from experience. The role of flax in fighting all forms of cancer is fairly well established. More specifically, many studies now show that men who consume about 40 grammes of milled flaxseed every day have a reduced risk for prostate cancer. The studies also show that the clinically detectable prostate cancers that do emerge tend not to spread and are more easily treated after exposure to flaxseed.

Dr Joiner-Bey urged Irish men to make their voice heard on this issue and to push for change in the area of prostate screening. 'It shouldn't be about "he who shouts loudest". This is about protecting and caring for people, irrespective of what sex they are.'

Centre of Excellence

Many people are looking to the area of complementary and integrated (combining alternative and orthodox medical approaches) therapies in the fight against all forms of cancer, including prostate. Take the Irish Centre for Integrated Medicine, for instance. Nestled away in Naas, County Dublin, the ICIM, it could be argued, is set up and ready to go as a dedicated prostate screening centre for the whole country. Why? Because it takes one of the biggest fears out of the whole process: it has found a way to do away with the dreaded DRE!

Dr Felipe Reitz heads up the centre. Reitz has what you could describe as an eclectic approach to the business of medicine. This approach is in keeping with the stated objective of the centre, which is to identify the root of the complaint using conventional diagnosis and to provide, where appropriate, a natural medical solution.

On the issue of prostate screening, Reitz pulls no punches: 'The relatively poor survival rate for prostate cancer can, in large part, be attributed to the fragmentation and protraction of the diagnosis services, which is not in accordance with best practice.'

OK, so what does he propose? 'First of all, you need to understand that just one test or examination is often not good enough for something like prostate cancer. The more medical tools we use, the better,' says Reitz.

True to his word, Reitz has introduced a One-Stop Prostate Assessment, which has five key elements:

§ questionnaire and consultation;

§ uroflowmetry (tests for blockages in the urine stream);

§ urine analysis;

§ ultrasound examination; and

§ a prostate-specific antigen reading.

And everything is done within an hour. That's *one* hour!

'The primary goal of this detailed assessment is risk reduction,' says Reitz. 'Early detection is an approach that promotes vigilance for signs and symptoms that may be indicative of early disease. It is based on the premise that [prostate cancer] is easier to treat and cure if it is detected early.'

My God! The man seems to be singing from my hymn sheet. He says that the immediate results of the tests allow the man to be screened and referred on to a specialist at a much faster rate than is possible at the moment. (Under the current system, a similar case could take up to nine months to process – and at a considerably higher cost.) Reitz also claims that this five-pronged approach yields an accuracy rate of at least 95 percent, compared to 70 percent from a PSA test alone. Them's good odds.

He rattles off a few recent statistics to frame the seriousness of the current situation:

§ The average number of prostate-cancer cases per year in Ireland is 1,371 (or 14 percent of total cancers);

§ As many as 519 men die from prostate cancer each year (that's 13 percent of the total);

§ The largest increase in cancer numbers was in cancer of the prostate, which increased by an average of 7.6 percent per year, from 1,089 cases in 1994 to 1,824 cases in 2001.

OK, so what can a patient expect from a visit to the Irish Centre for Integrated Medicine? 'When the patient comes to the centre, we go through a specific risk-assessment questionnaire, where a symptom evaluation is made. We check current medication, family history, etc. So, in general, this specific questionnaire gives us a better indication of the clinical conditions that may be present,' says Reitz.

'After the questionnaire, we perform an ultrasound; the patient must present with a full bladder so that we can observe both kidneys and measure the capacity of the bladder. We then conduct the uroflowmetry. This calculates the degree of any potential obstruction, by measuring the volume against time in the urine flow.

'Then, what I consider the important breakthrough in the whole process: the ultrasound. As well as measuring possible urine residue in the bladder, the ultrasound is the replacement for the digital rectal examination, the invasive procedure that turns most men off even the idea of having a prostate examination.

'I have seen many patients here, along with my colleague Dr Gaier, and all patients are more comfortable with our system, especially because it is not an invasive procedure,' says Reitz. 'You see, even for me as a doctor, it is not nice to give patients a physical examination.'

When all the information has been gathered, the next step is to conduct a PSA test. 'All the test results are put together and are presented to the patient. We then write up a report for the patient's doctor or consultant. With all these results together, we can find prostate disorders much earlier and eliminate the chances of being too late to intervene.'

Statistically, 1 in every 6 men will develop prostate cancer and, in the next thirteen years – if we don't do anything to counter the problem – this proportion will rise to become more than 1 in 3. The situation would appear to be critical.

'I am sure that the prostate assessment carried out here at the centre is the best chance Ireland ever had to adopt the first National Prostate Screening Programme,' says Reitz. 'This would do a number of things: it would facilitate doctors in referring any suspicious cases for screening; it would ease the minds of patients if they know that there is a national programme in place; and it would lead the way on prostate-cancer prevention.'

It's an enticing prospect: the centre

is there, the equipment is there, the expertise is there, the will and the desire is there . . .

(You can contact the Irish Centre of Integrated Medicine on 045 844 819, or you can get more information about them on www.icim.ie.)

The Natural Approach

There are many natural remedies indicated for prostate problems, and one of the main advantages is that they can be taken safely in conjunction with medication prescribed by your doctor. (You do have to check this with your doctor, however.)

A recent report in the respected medical journal *Urology* found that saw palmetto can 'significantly ease symptoms of BPH' (benign prostatic hypertrophy – enlargement of the prostate). According to the study, symptoms improved dramatically in more than 20 percent of men after just two months, and in 46 percent after six months. Saw Palmetto is a powerful herb which works by altering hormone levels. It also packs a hell of a punch when it comes to reducing inflammation.

Nettle root is also indicated by naturopaths for prostate problems because of its ability to reduce the severity of symptoms and slow the march of BPH. According to the *Guide to Vitamins, Minerals and Supplements* (published by the *Reader's Digest*), the active ingredi-

111

ent in both saw palmetto and nettle root is a little kicker called betasitosterol. This is also available in its pure form as a dietary supplement.

When it comes to vitamins, vitamin E seems to be effective in tackling prostate problems. Finnish scientists conducted a study that involved as many as 30,000 men (who were also classified as smokers). The scientists discovered that those who took vitamin E were almost a third less likely to develop prostate cancer.

Finally, the nutrient with the best chance of battling BPH is zinc. It has been shown to reduce the size of the gland and ease the symptoms of BPH.

Acupuncture

This ancient Oriental medical art involves the stimulation of various 'meridian' points on the body, to get the juices flowing again. The Chinese believe that meridians (or energy pathways) trace specific patterns and routes in the body and that, by stimulating or depressing these, you can affect the health of related areas.

According to traditional Chinese medicine, prostate cancer, or any abnormal enlargement of the prostate, is mostly due to dodgy kidney qi. Qi is the term the Chinese use for 'vital energy'. They believe that qi is in every living organism and is the source of all movement and flux in the universe, and that everything is connected in some way to this shimmering web of energy. (For more on this, read *The Web That Has No Weaver* by Ted Kaptchuk.)

Chinese medicine holds that when blood passing through the kidney becomes static, or blocked, due to toxic accumulation in the 'lower Jiao' (the abdomen), there can be an interruption in the flow of qi and an enlargement of the prostate. The treatment, therefore, is to revitalise or increase qi circulation in the kidneys and the blood.

Medical studies would appear to back up the effectiveness of this approach. Once qi has been restored, patients begin to feel an improvement in symptoms, including weak urinary stream, broken sleep, lower back pain and depression.

Watchful Waiting

Ask any person in the street what 'watchful waiting' is and he will probably tell you that it is simply 'doing nothing'. And he wouldn't be far wrong.

Watchful waiting is a much-practised 'approach' adopted by the medical profession in the 'treatment' of prostate problems. But it's an approach that Professor Fred Stephens feels can cause confusion. He has gone on the record with his concerns: 'This strategy can be hard for patients and their families to understand, as we are used to being told that early detection and treatment of cancer is essential for cure.'

Writing in his book *Prostate Cancer*, Stephens says that a patient exhibiting signs of prostate cancer could be suffering from a 'latent cancer'. This is a malignancy that can lie dormant or progress very slowly 'without bothering the patient before a more rapid health problem, or old age, takes his life'.

Watchful waiting is also known as the 'observation or surveillance' approach. It means that no active treatment is engaged in until symptoms appear. Doctors are known to favour this approach because it can spare a man a difficult invasive technique, like surgery or radiation – which is fair enough. However, there is a downside to this 'treatment' option: you may lose the chance to control the disease before it spreads. You are also postponing treatment to an age, and a stage, when it may be more difficult for the man to tolerate.

Another possible disadvantage of watchful waiting lies in the fact that it increases the anxiety rate of the men who are being 'watched'. Some men do not want the worry of not knowing what could be growing inside them and would much prefer an invasive investigation.

In fairness, many men who choose watchful waiting live for years without developing significant signs of the disease. A number of studies have found that there is not that much difference in the life expectancy of men who undergo surgery and those who are merely observed through watchful waiting.

There's only one problem – and it comes in the form of a new study which has been published in the prestigious *New England Journal of Medicine*. This study says that prostate-cancer patients who have surgery are more likely to be alive after ten years than men who opt for watchful waiting.

How so? Because the men who chose surgery were much less likely to see their cancers spread to other organs.

Radical Prostatectomy

We have to look to the US for concrete comparisons when it comes to the treatment of prostate cancer. And here's how they've been doing it: in the early 1990s, roughly 50 percent of prostate patients were treated by surgery, 30 percent by radiation, and 20 percent by watchful waiting. In Europe, by contrast, watchful waiting constitutes the standard treatment for asymptomatic presentation of the condition (no visible sign of prostate disease).

Surgery has been a very popular way to treat prostate cancer in the States in recent years. The number of men receiving what is known as a radical prostatectomy has increased six-fold – and the increase has been seen in all age groups.

Radical prostatectomy involves the complete removal of the prostate and all nearby tissue. The surgeon can go in through incisions in a number of different areas. In a retro-pubic prostatectomy, the prostate is reached through an incision in the lower abdomen; in a perineal prostatectomy, the approach is through an area known as the perineum, the space between the scrotum and the anus.

When the surgeon gets to the site, the section of urethra that runs through the prostate is cut away, as is the neck of the bladder and, with it, some sphincter muscle. Hey, it's not called a 'radical' prostatectomy for nothing! It's a complicated and demanding procedure which usually requires that the patient is knocked out with a general anaesthesia. Anything from two to four hours is the norm for this surgery. Patients are hospitalised for about three days and need to wear a tube (catheter) to drain urine for between ten days and three weeks.

According to the US Federal Consumer Information Center (an organisation which has investigated the area of prostate problems and how they are treated in America), about 5 to 10 percent of patients experience surgery-related complications such as bleeding, infection or cardiopulmonary (heart-valve) problems. There is also a small risk of death from this surgery. It is less for men who are young and healthy than for men who are older and frail, however.

Prostatectomy can also carry the risk of debilitating long-term problems, notably urinary incontinence, stool incontinence and sexual impotence.

At one time, prostatectomy almost invariably resulted in sexual problems. Today, however, the risk of impotence may be reduced by a procedure called nerve-sparing. This technique carefully avoids cutting or snatching two bundles of nerves and blood vessels that run close to the surface of the prostate gland and are needed to help achieve and maintain an erection.

The problem is that nerve-sparing surgery is not possible for everyone. Sometimes the cancer is too large or is located too close to the nerves. Even with nerve-sparing surgery, many men, especially older men, become impotent.

Most men undergoing this procedure will lose a degree of sexual function. Depending on age, extent of disease and type of surgery, the chances of impotence vary widely – somewhere between 20 and 90 percent.

Radiation Therapy

Radiation therapy uses high-energy X-rays, either beamed from a machine or emitted by radioactive seeds specially implanted in the prostate to kill cancer cells.

When prostate cancer is localised (confined to one area), radiation therapy is a definite option and a real alternative to surgery.

There are problems with this form of therapy. Because the radiation beam passes through normal tissues, including the rectum, bladder and intestines, on its way to the prostate, it can kill some healthy cells. With newer techniques, side effects can be lessened. State-of-the-art radiation 'guns' can be focused more precisely, while computer technology is now allowing radiation oncologists to be more target-specific when it comes to isolating a specific part of the patient's anatomy.

When the cancer has spread beyond the prostate gland itself, it can be beyond the reach of local treatments like surgery and radiation therapy. That is when doctors look to hormone therapy as a treatment option.

The logic behind hormone therapy is clear: it takes the fight to prostate cancer by cutting off the supply of male hormones, such as testosterone, which encourage the growth of the cancer. One of the more crude hormone controls is the complete removal of the testicles, which are the main source of testosterone. Another, less crude, method is medication (discussed below).

Although doctors never use the word 'cure' in the same breath as 'hormone therapy', this approach does have an important role to play in relation to prostate-cancer management. Hormone therapy can shrink or halt the worst ravages of the disease, often deferring the more advanced form of the cancer for years.

Hormone therapy is not without its side effects. According to the US Federal Consumer Information Centre, surgical castration (orchiectomy) or medical castration (hormonal drug therapy) can produce a 'striking response'. Both approaches cause tumours and lymph nodes to shrink and PSA levels to fall, but both can also cause hot flushes, impotence and a general loss of interest in sex. Medical castration can cause breast enlargement and an increased risk of cardiovascular problems, including heart attack and stroke.

Unfortunately, hormone therapy for metastatic disease (cancer that has spread from the original site) works only for a limited time. Remissions typically occur in two to three years. Eventually, cancer cells that do not feed off testosterone begin to flourish, and the growth of the cancer resumes.

Cryosurgery

Cryosurgery uses liquid nitrogen to freeze and kill prostate-cancer cells. Thin metal cryo-probes are inserted through the skin of the perineum into the prostate. Liquid nitrogen in the cryo-probes forms an ice ball that freezes the prostate-cancer cells. As the cells thaw, they rupture.

During cryosurgery, a warming catheter is inserted through the penis to protect the urethra and, as a consequence, incontinence is seldom a problem. However, impotence can result because the adjacent nerve bundles usually freeze.

Drugs Used to Treat Prostate Problems

One of the main ways to take the fight to prostate cancer is to drop a little napalm bomb into the mix. This comes in the form of various chemotherapy drugs, which blitz anything that gets in their way, including the rogue cells, of course. This approach is not without its side effects. You are probably aware of the main ones, which include nausea, hair loss and all manner of sores. But, for some, these indignities are worth the pain.

There are many drugs on the market that are used to treat prostate cancers. A very random selection includes the following:

§ *Doxorubicin* (names change depending on the country in which they are launched), which is classified as an anti-tumour antibiotic. It works a bit like a pack of maurading ninjas, getting in under cover of darkness and playing havoc with the mechanism of the cancer cell by damaging the nuclei.

§ Another interesting drug goes by the name of *Vinblastine*. It's an antieoplastic (think Semtex!), which draws its effectiveness from blowing cells apart! Get this: it's derived from the Madagascar periwinkle!

§ *Etoposide* takes a more measured approach. It kills off the cancer cells by slowing down the processes by which they replicate.

§ *Paclitaxel* is a member of the powerful Taxane group. This drug works by attaching itself, limpet-like, to the scaffolding of the cancer cell, thereby causing the cell to crumble.

There is one more drug that I want to draw your attention to. It goes by the name of *Prostap* and is made by Wyeth Pharmaceuticals. It is proving very effective. It was launched in 2004 (a relative baby in pharmaceutical terms) and was designed specifically to deal with aggressive, late-stage prostate cancers; in other words, a heavy hitter!

Prostap is structured in such a way as to knock the fight right out of prostate-cancer cells by attacking their very life-force: testosterone. It does this in a roundabout sort of way, by first targeting the leuteinising hormone which feeds

121

testosterone: a bit like cutting the posse off at the pass!

Things got a little better for Wyeth and Prostap in 2008. So impressed were medical scientists with the efficacy and progress of the drug that it has been upgraded considerably, to the point where it is now at a level at which it can be used to treat virtually all stages of the disease, from locally advanced to metastatic spread.

16

If Not Now, When?

A German by the name of Eckhart Tolle has managed to do what few people have done in the past: he has got people to focus on the *now*!

Back in 1999, with the help of the good folk at Hodder and Stoughton, he published a little book with a big message. The message was simply this: live for the moment!

I know what you're thinking: it's hardly original, is it? True, but somebody needed to say it again, because most of us have lost the ability to live for the here and now.

The question has to be asked: what are our lives about? The way we live our lives seems to be, in large part, looking back at what has gone before and looking forward to what is yet to come. Both are illusions. The past is gone. The future may never happen. Essentially, there is no tomorrow.

But if tomorrow comes around, you can only experience it in the now! Enslaved by memories and enticed by anticipation is no way to live, because neither is real.

Tolle has said a few things that are particularly relevant to people who suddenly find themselves in the grip of a life-changing event. He said: 'Death is a stripping away of all that is not you. The secret of life is to "die before you die" – and find that there is no death.'

And then he asked one of the most incisive questions that anyone can ask: 'If not now, when?' It's an approach that Alexander Ager can identify with.

Last year, this Dublin-based technician was diagnosed with prostate cancer. His story is important for many reasons, but primarily because it illustrates what happens when you are not proactive in relation to this condition.

At sixty years of age, Alexander was at the top of his game. He worked as a trainer for the giant telecommunications firm Ericsson, and he loved his job.

'No day was the same,' he says. 'One morning you could wake up in Capetown; the next, Paris. I got to travel the world and meet wonderful, motivated people every day.'

Ericsson is one of the more progressive companies to work for. As well as paying well, it also has a good health policy.

After suffering a few bouts of illness and, occasionally, passing blood in his urine, Alexander decided that it was time for a visit to the company doctor. After a number of protracted PSA tests and a biopsy, he was finally diagnosed with cancer of the prostate.

'Honestly, when I heard the word "cancer", I didn't hear another thing after that. My mind was in a fog. I knew that the doctor was talking to me, but I couldn't focus on a word he said.'

This is typical of many people diagnosed with cancer, particularly men. With the dawning realisation comes the inevitable numbness.

In time, he was taken through his options. He could have surgery, or radiation therapy. 'Surgery. Radiation. They were just words to me. Words I was only vaguely aware of. I had no idea of the implications. I was in no position to make such a radical choice. I didn't have enough knowledge. But the doctors said the choice was mine to make,' says Alexander.

Limiting The Damage

He opted for radiation therapy, simply because he was told that this would allow him to be sexually active afterwards.

Impotence can be one of the big side effects of invasive prostate treatments. Alexander was justifiably concerned about this and wanted to limit the damage as much as he could.

'People might say that I had reached a point in my life [he is over sixty] where sex shouldn't be as important to me as it once was. Fair enough. But the thing is, it is still very important to me and my wife. I have a wife who is fifteen years younger than me. I have an eight-year-old boy. I want life to go on as it always has, and that shouldn't be too much to ask.'

That was the theory. The reality proved to be a little different, however.

At times, he was passing so much blood that he had to wear his wife's sanitary towels. At other times, he was on so much medication that he didn't know if he was coming or going.

'I didn't handle the whole radiation thing very well. The effects were terrible. The mood swings were incredible. I found myself bursting into tears all the time. I was sapped of all energy. By the end of session thirty-seven, I could barely crawl up the stairs on all fours. It was devastating.'

He says that what kept him sane during the heavyweight treatment was that little oasis called ARC House. Everything about cancer – the long-term implications, the side effects, the psychological fallout – are explained in easy-to-understand terms.

'Without ARC, I don't think I would have been able to pull through,' says Alexander. 'They made me and my wife feel much more comfortable about tackling the condition. They were always there for me when I needed to cry, or fly off the handle. They are simply incredible people. I would advise anybody newly diagnosed with any form of cancer to seek out the people in ARC House. It could make all the difference.'

Locked-in Feelings

He has another piece of advice for men who develop prostate cancer: tell the wife!

'When I first heard, I decided to keep it to myself for a while. I didn't want to tell her. I didn't want to worry her. But she will find out eventually, and sooner than you think. Then, the shock and the hurt can be all the more damaging.'

It's an approach that leading cancer counsellor Joel Nathan agrees with. He says that you may feel that you want to protect those around you by staying silent. But keeping your feelings locked in will not only increase your own distress, it will add to their unease as well.

'If no one knows how you feel, they are likely to imagine the worst. Instead of protecting them, you may have to deal with their feelings in addition to your own,' says Nathan. 'You may find the process of calming others part of your duty, but you need to maintain your independence and your autonomy, so remind yourself who is the patient, who needs rest and whose life is on the line.'

Alexander Ager feels that one of the major problems with the whole issue of prostate cancer is lack of awareness. 'I was like most men . . . I didn't really know what the prostate was, what it was for, or where you would find it. Men are different from women in that sense: women are a lot more proactive when it comes to their health and looking after themselves. They build up a relationship with their doctor, much more so than men. And, I feel, that it is this relationship that can help in the long term.'

A New Rhythm

A year after the nightmare began with his positive diagnosis for prostate cancer, Alexander is beginning to settle into a new rhythm.

'I feel I'm getting over the whole thing. I still have to get up during the night and I still have to take a load of medication. I'm on medication to improve my calcium because, at one stage, my bones were so weak that I suffered a prolapsed disc in my back. I'm also on tablets to keep my moods stable. The good news is that I'm going on holiday with my wife for the first time in two years, and I feel this is an important step forward for me, not just physically but emotionally as well.'

In theory, he agrees with the principle of screening for prostate cancer. In practice, however, he found it more than a little invasive. 'I honestly feel that if it wasn't for the DRE, more men would happily have their prostate checked out. The first few times it was performed on me, I felt affronted. Yeah, that's the word. It was a little like an invasion of me as a person. When I began to understand what the doctor was looking for, I knew why I had to go through the procedure. But, I have to tell you, it was never easy. It wasn't painful physically. There was pressure, certainly. But more than that, there was indignity.'

The indignity was removed, in part, by the 'Male Cancer' classes he attended in ARC House, which included meditation sessions. At times, they were his salvation. And they helped him echo something Eckhart Tolle said: 'When you focus within and feel the inner body, you immediately become still and present, as you are withdrawing consciousness from the mind.'

Sometimes, it helps to think of other things. 'Prostate cancer has done one thing for me: it has helped me live more in the moment. When I wake up in the morning, I now say: "Great, it's another day." I feel I want to embrace the day. Before that I would have been just like everyone else and taken the day for granted. Now, I'm seeing things and appreciating things a lot better.'

According to Eckhart Tolle, this is a marvellous, healing approach. He says: 'Use your senses fully. Be where you are. Look around. Just look, don't interpret. See the light, shapes, colours, textures. Be aware of the silent presence of each thing. Be aware of the space that allows everything to be. Listen to the sounds; don't judge them. Listen to the silence underneath the sounds. Touch something – anything – and feel and acknowledge its being. Observe the rhythm of your breathing; feel the air flowing in and out, feel the life-energy inside your body. Allow everything to be, within and without. Allow the 'is-ness' of all things. Move deeply into the now.'

17

Twin Tracks

On the same day we spoke to Alexander Ager, consultant urologist Dr Thomas Lynch was on a train travelling to Galway. There are parallels between the two men's experiences of prostate cancer, except that they are coming at the problem from different sides of the track. One is acutely aware of the prostate because it almost killed him; the other is acutely aware of it because he tries to prevent it from killing.

Dr Lynch is one of the physicians used on the most recent Irish prostate-awareness campaign, a campaign spearheaded by pharmaceutical firm AstraZeneca. He is a strong advocate of raising awareness when it comes to the prostate gland and the potential damage it can cause. A dapper, chatty, friendly man, he wants to send the message that men need to take charge of this situation and be proactive when it comes to their health.

'Many men with early prostate cancer are unlikely to have symptoms,' he said. 'Therefore, it is important that men must be prostate-aware.'

He feels that part of the problem here lies in the fact that symptoms of actual prostate cancer can be very similar to signs of an enlarged prostate (benign prostatic hyperplasia), a condition which will cause considerable discomfort if left unchecked, but will not kill you.

However, the problem is that most men wouldn't know a symptom of prostate cancer if it came up and bit them on the ass!

In fact, a startling 52 percent of men surveyed as part of the AstraZeneca awareness campaign were unable to identify any of the symptoms of prostate cancer. The situation is further complicated when you consider that, although the vast majority of men know that they have to get along to their GP for investigation, only 47 percent actually do so. That leaves a huge number of Irish men who are putting themselves needlessly at risk.

Dr Lynch, as part of the awareness campaign, advised men to pay a visit to their GP if they are worried about signs of prostate cancer. But as the survey shows that most men are unaware of the signs, symptoms, location or function of the prostate, there are no early warning bells going off, only late ones.

Dr Lynch says that if prostate cancer is present and is localised (in other words, if it hasn't spread), there are treatment options which can have a positive outcome.

In other words: catch the thing early.

Unfortunately, though, we're not doing that!

Out of Control

The situation is getting out of control. The latest figures show that there has been a major increase in the number of reported cases of prostate cancer. Let's take one year: 2001. In that year, a whopping 2,100 new cases of prostate cancer were diagnosed in Irish men. In the same year, 543 men died of the condition.

It could be argued, at this point, that men aren't capable of taking health matters into their own hands, and that no amount of awareness campaigns will get the message to hit home. The question could be justifiably asked: how many more men have to die before something is done to rectify the situation?

Meanwhile, back on the train to Galway, Dr Lynch is on the phone, discussing the merits and demerits of screening for prostate cancer. 'We don't have the full facts and figures to say that prostate screening would work. There a study going on at the moment in the UK which should give us a few more pointers in the right direction.'

How long will it take for that study to be completed, I ask him.

'A number of years.'

Men are dropping like flies because of

this condition, and we're still crunching numbers!

The train continues clattering on down the track towards Galway, and Dr Lynch's phone signal is fading in and out of coverage; but he can still make out my growing sense of frustration with the argument.

'Look,' he says, trying to bring some evidence-based sense to the position, 'I'm not saying no to screening, but I'm not saying yes either. We simply have to wait and see what the best practice is. Right now, the best practice seems to be to do nothing.

'Three-quarters of the men who come back with elevated PSA tests will have nothing wrong with them. Well, they won't have prostate cancer; it'll be a combination of other things. Screening then opens up the whole area of "the worried well", where men will be anxious for no reason at all.

'My advice to men would be: go get yourself checked out. Don't wait for an invitation. Be proactive.'

He does feel, however, that when it comes to being proactive, men would do well to ape their female betters.

'It's true, men don't have the same relationship with their doctors that women do; and they are less good at carrying out advice than their female counterparts. On top of this, when it comes to active health campaigns, women have surpassed their male counterparts. That's why we have a breast screening programme in this country, and that's why a cervical screening programme has recently been introduced as well.'

Men need help in this regard.

And they need it now.

18

Meetings of the Mind

Lisbon. A late-evening haze is settling in over the city as we drive to our destination: the sixth European Cancer Conference.

The great and the good are gathered together in the ancient Portuguese city to discuss the very latest findings on prostate cancer, with particular emphasis on screening.

The mood is strangely upbeat. Normally, at events like this, people are jostling for intellectual bragging rights and flashing the 'old school tie'. Lisbon, for some reason, is different. There seems to be a pervading let's-get-things-done approach.

In the lobby of the ostentatious Hotel Lisboa, large amounts of sticky buns are being consumed, together with gallons of fine coffee.

Over in one corner, there is a man who looks for all the world like a mad professor: resplendent in flyaway Einstein hair and white socks. If you are looking for scatty genius, the socks are always a dead giveaway!

I sidle over to him.

Turns out that he is a professor – a professor of urology, to be exact. I eventually get around to telling him that I'm doing a book on prostate screening.

'Ah, screening,' he says, looking into the half-distance and pulling out of the air one of the most succinct summaries of the standpoints on this particular issue that I have ever heard.

'There are very definite arguments for and against,' he said, and then he bullet-pointed them for me.

Arguments For

§ The PSA test saves lives;

§ The test can detect tumours at an early stage, when they are easily treatable;

§ Men with advanced prostate cancer can also benefit from PSA screening if it leads to immediate treatment;

§ PSA is more reliable than digital rectal screening, and there is no better alternative available at the moment;

§ A false positive may cause anxiety (one of the big arguments from the anti-screening camp),

but it can be worth it if it
leads to a satisfactory outcome.

He paused for a beat, weighing up the
counter-argument, gathered himself, and
then launched into it.

Arguments Against

§ It has never been proven that
PSA screening actually saves
lives;

§ Detecting an early-stage tumour
doesn't necessarily mean that it
needs to be treated. Some
prostate tumours grow so slowly
that they will never show symptoms or become life-threatening,
particularly for older men with
a lower life expectancy;

§ Men are subjected to treatments
with potential side effects that
could seriously affect quality
of life - things like impotence
and lack of sexual desire;

§ High PSA levels are not necessarily an indication of cancer.
Instead, they could be linked to
an enlarged prostate, which is a
normal part of getting older for
most men. What is needed is a
test that can determine not only
whether a man has prostate

cancer, but how aggressive the tumour is;

§ False-positive readings are a major problem. They can lead to unnecessary biopsies, which can, in turn, result in complications like infections and bleeding.

Dodging the Dilemma

By the time I pull myself away from the Prof, the conference is under way. One of the big arguments against introducing a prostate screening programme is that we may end up with a small army of men who qualify as 'worried well'.

It's an issue that Professor Fritz Schroder addressed at the conference; and he would appear to have a way out of the dilemma.

He said the way forward is to involve men in the process as much as possible. He believes that it's vital to arm them with as much information as possible.

'Men deserve to hear the full facts before being asked to undergo a test that could reveal prostate cancer,' said Prof Schroder, who hails from the Netherlands.

He went as far as to say that it was 'unethical' to apply the test without first making sure men understood the implications of a positive or negative result.

Let's set the scene, in simple terms

The PSA test looks for chemical markers in the blood. High levels of these markers suggest that the man may have prostate cancer.

However, two-thirds of men with elevated PSA levels don't actually have the disease. It could just be that they have a simple infection or an inflammation of the prostate. In addition, some men who have completely normal PSA readings do turn out to have cancer.

'Powerful, early diagnostic tests cannot be withheld from well-informed men,' said the professor. 'The emphasis here, however, has to be on "well-informed".'

The conference heard that, in the US, widespread PSA testing has vastly increased the number of prostate cancers detected, but very many of these are slow-growing tumours in elderly men and are unlikely to pose a direct threat to life.

This said, many men decided to go ahead with invasive treatment options anyway. There are inherent dangers with this. Because the prostate gland lies just under the bladder, it is situated close to a number of tissues and other vital areas that are important for normal bladder and sexual function. Consequently, it is difficult for surgeons or radiologists to avoid damaging these sensitive areas.

The conference heard of one study that

followed a number of patients who had their prostate gland removed. After eighteen months, 60 percent were impotent, 8 percent had complete urinary incontinence and 40 percent had occasional genito-urinary problems of one sort or another.

Paris. After we negotiate a packed Charles de Gaulle Airport, we pile into a taxi and head straight for the 2005 European Urology Conference. Some of the world's foremost urologists are gathered in the French capital to discuss the issue of prostate cancer and how best to manage the condition. There are a few pointers that we can take from the conference, but not many.

The role for true prostate screening is not fully proven. To be 'fully proven' would require absolute proof that screening will bring about a direct decrease in the death rate from this particular form of the disease. Trials, in this regard, are ongoing.

Running counter to this, the American Cancer Society, the American Radiological Association and the American Urological Association, the conference heard, recommend early detection with an annual DRE and PSA, beginning at the age of fifty for all men.

In relation to DRE, the conference heard that more cancers are detected with the use of DRE and PSA than with either examination alone. If more men undergo a PSA (the less invasive form of testing), abnormal DRE examinations are much less common.

cPSA (or complex PSA) is a new and more sensitive test that aims to detect abnormalities in the prostate gland. The conference was told that, as a single test for screening, cPSA may reduce the number of unnecessary prostate biopsies.

We left Paris much as we had arrived: we knew that studies were ongoing in relation to prostate screening; we knew that detecting prostate cancer earlier in its life cycle could lead to improved outcome; and we knew that DRE in association with PSA was always going to give us a clearer picture.

From Paris to Cork! Tracking down a killer can be a tiresome business . . .

19

Balancing Act

A Tale of Two Doctors

The little Cork fishing village of Carrigaline has on its best bib 'n' tucker. Brand-new boats bob, and tiny sailships shimmer in the white glare of an early-morning sun. The air whipping in off the Atlantic Ocean stings the lungs and brings with it the promise of a fresh start. This is where Dr Sean Dunphy has made his home, and there's nowhere else on earth he'd rather be.

On the one hand, Sean Dunphy is your typical GP: he operates out of a custom-built surgery and enjoys a healthy private practice. On the other hand, he's also one of the more progressive physicians, combining traditional treatment options with the more complementary approaches like colour therapy in a bid to find the best solution for his patients.

He is friendliness personified and, whenever you are lucky enough to find yourself in his part of the world, you are greeted like a prodigal returned.

At the mention of the word 'prostate', the doctor clicks into gear. 'If a man in the "at risk" group (circa fifty and up) came to see me with something unrelated, like a sore throat, for instance, I would have a tendency to approach the subject of a prostate check,' says Dr Dunphy.

He feels that once the issue is out in the open, you are 'pushing against an open door'. 'I don't believe most men have a problem with having their prostate checked. At least, that's my experience. A PSA test is easy to handle and process, while the DRE is, by now, a routine enough procedure.'

Dr Dunphy examines the prostate as a matter of course in presenting male patients. But he's the exception to the rule. Why?

'Because time has become a precious commodity,' he says.

'The way the system is structured now, it's a lot easier just to write a prescription than pop somebody up on a couch for a full examination. If you do that with everyone you think might benefit from it, you are adding an hour or two to your day.'

It's conveyor-belt medicine, folks: get 'em in and get 'em out. One of the chief complaints patients make now is that their doctor doesn't seem to have enough time just to talk to them. It's not the doctor's fault; it's certainly not the patient's fault. The fault lies with the system. If you spend your day simply treating a set of symptoms in a regimented, evidence-based way, pretty soon you can forget that there is a real person behind the symptoms.

Dr Dunphy feels that we have certainly progressed in our medical knowledge and in the way we treat patients. But there is a flip side. 'I feel that the practical side of medicine has been watered down a little. It's practical to examine people who you feel need to be examined, but many of us don't make the time to do that now.'

Hard to Interpret

OK, taking on board all the time-consuming considerations, would he still be in favour of screening for prostate cancer?

'Yes! I would welcome a screening programme. There are two sides to this story, however. The governing bodies feel that it can be hard to interpret prostate results and that it can create a lot of anxiety among the patient population.

'This said, I feel that it would create a little bit of balance. Women are being screened for things like breast cancer. Why should men be any different when it comes to putting their health first? The answer is: they shouldn't!

'Men are usually the breadwinners in the family, and it makes sense to look after them. I don't think there is a GP in this country who wouldn't be willing to look after men if a screening programme was put in place.'

Well said. But screening takes time and, in medicine, time is money. Who is going to pay for all this?

Dr Dunphy is well aware of the rather clichéd view of men, in that they would prefer to be doing anything other than sitting in their GP's waiting room. But he feels that the problem is not insurmountable.

'By and large, men don't like going to their doctor; we'll take this as a given. But when they do eventually find their way into the surgery, they want a complete M.O.T. They want the works!'

The first step is to get men into surgery. And the best way to do that is to offer them something worthwhile. Something like a screening programme; something that could save their lives.

The Doctor as Patient

Dr Seamus Monely was a great physician. All his patients said so. For years, he worked as one of the country's top gynaecologists. His life was devoted to looking after the health and well-being of women. So it is perhaps a great irony that he should have been diagnosed with a disease that is the curse of men who fail to look after their own health.

A number of years ago, at the age of fifty-nine, he began noticing the worrying signs; little pointers that snag on the consciousness and refuse to let go. 'I was getting up more often during the night to go to the toilet,' he said, 'and then, after a while, the stinging became quite severe.'

He tried to push the nagging thoughts to the back of his mind; and that's when his own surgery nurses stepped in. 'They insisted that I get a PSA,' he said.

The test came back positive. 'To be honest, I just thought it was the sign of a kidney infection.'

It wasn't. To cut a long story short, between the jigs and the reels, Dr Monely was diagnosed with prostate cancer. That was the bad news. The 'good' news was that it hadn't spread. For now.

He was booked into St Luke's Hospital in Dublin for radiotherapy. He spent seven weeks there and underwent as many as thirty-five treatments. His PSA levels came right down. All was well.

For the next couple of years, Dr Monely tried, as best he could, to get on with his life. Then, disaster struck again. Prostate cancer is not something you can take your eye off. Let your guard down for a second, and it will decide to pay you another visit. That's exactly what happened in Dr Monely's case.

He started experiencing pains in his neck. Bone scans showed that he had little specks on his spine. On closer inspection, it was discovered that a tumour on his spine had broken his neck. The problem was so acute that it was quite possible that he could have killed himself shaving!

An MRI test showed that he had four compressions on his spine, which meant that he was on the verge of paralysis. Session after session of chemotherapy followed.

He pulled through, and today he is still fighting the good fight. But he is a little confused. 'I don't know why this disease chose me. I was never sick a day in my life. I didn't smoke or drink. I had a normal diet. Genetically, there wasn't anything in my family that would have predisposed me to the condition.'

As with a lot of cancers, it was just fate. The ability of the body's cells to divide and replicate themselves comes at a price; for some, the price is just a little too high.

Having been through the torment of prostate cancer, Dr Monely has one piece of advice for other men. 'Start looking for it before you are fifty. Prostate cancer is no longer an old-man's disease.' He is also very much in favour of a screening programme for men to detect the condition – a condition that responds well if it is caught early.

There is a certain bravery about Dr Monely. You get the impression that he is up for the fight. He doesn't appear to have any time for self-pity. He puts things into context: 'A coward dies a thousand times, a brave man only once.'

Dr Monely's case is important for a number of reasons. It goes to show that even someone with his clinical skills can be caught off guard by this disease.

It goes to show that you can't take your eyes off this condition because, just when you thought you had it beaten, it bounces back. It goes to show that certain forms of this scourge can spread quickly and aggressively and can travel great distances in the body.

What is also clear from this case is that prostate cancer is absolutely no respecter of age, standing or reputation.

20

Personalities and the Prostate

Most sports fans will be familiar with the image of the great Pelé rising high above the Italian defence to power home a header into the bottom corner of the goal in the 1970 World Cup final. It is one of the most famous TV clips of soccer, and is regularly rolled out to illustrate the magic of the World Cup.

Pelé is sitting in front of me now in a Dublin hotel. He is on one of those whistle-stop tours of European cities, promoting men's health issues and, in particular, sexual health.

The good people at pharmaceutical giant Pfizer are using the legend to endorse the sexual-health benefits of Viagra. They couldn't have picked a better role model.

The Merrion Hotel, just across the street from Government Buildings, is filled to bursting point with a mixture of sports and health journalists. Pelé is at the top table, surrounded by slightly stuffy medics, who are there to deliver facts and figures, and to make sure we all fall into line with the evidence-based data. The great man, however, just wants to connect with the audience. He is engaging, articulate, funny. The unfortunate physicians are beginning to pale next to him, swamped by his sheer enthusiasm.

After the press conference, I manage to sneak a private interview with one of the greatest sporting heroes on the planet. Pretty quickly, our conversation turns to health screening for men.

I tell him that we don't yet have a screening programme to detect prostate cancer in Ireland.

He is genuinely shocked. 'When I was playing for the Brazilian soccer team, we had to undergo regular prostate examinations,' he tells me. 'Not just the blood test, but also the physical examination.'

'You had no choice. It was a requirement of the team management, so you just went with it. We never questioned it because we knew it was a measure designed to look after our health. We knew that this simple measure could one day save our lives.'

He is shocked at our lack of a screening programme because he classes Ireland as a 'very progressive' country, 'a rich country where health care shouldn't be something you have to bargain for'. His words.

He looks at me. For the first time that

day, his expression hardens. 'Listen, you have to organise the men of Ireland to shout about this. If they shout, they will be heard. If they do nothing, nothing will be done.'

The List Goes On

Personalities and prostate cancer seem to go hand in hand.

The list of prominent men who have been diagnosed with prostate cancer includes such dignitaries as former New York mayor Rudy Giuliani, former US Secretary of State Colin Powell, 'Stormin' Norman Schwarzkopf, publishing magnate Rupert Murdoch, golfer Arnold Palmer . . . and so it goes on.

Giuliani's cancer was discovered not long after his finest hour, following the Twin Towers outrage. Standing on the steps of New York's City Hall, he announced to the assembled masses that he had prostate cancer. He delivered the news with what watching journalists described as 'warmth, solemnity and confidence'.

'The bad news is that it's cancer,' he said. 'The good news is there are lots of possible options.'

Giuliani's physician, Dr Alexander Kirschenbaum, said that they had caught the disease in the very early stages, after the former mayor had been screened.

'Several of the samples – thank goodness not all, and not most – had indications of cancer,' said Giuliani.

According to one journalist who was present at the announcement, Giuliani tried to lighten the mood by claiming that the treatment he was about to undergo would in no way change his character.

'Will I have a sweeter disposition afterwards? No way. No way,' he joked.

The Barriers

Golfer Arnold Palmer also underwent treatment for prostate cancer, and he is well aware of the barriers that most men erect when it comes to identifying the condition.

'I guess most of us would rather not discuss cancer because we are all afraid we might be told we have it,' said Palmer in an interview on the Proactive health website.

'It's hard for people to even say the word [cancer], and that's the first obstacle you have to overcome when you are diagnosed with the disease. I think, once you understand a little more about it, you give more in-depth thought to how you are going to deal with it.'

Palmer was presented with a number of treatment options by his doctor. 'I chose the aggressive option,' Palmer said. 'I chose surgery, and I'm happy with that decision. I was fortunate to experience no side effects, other than the recovery period, which was, for me, rather lengthy.

I looked at it like this: if you're recovering from cancer, then you're in "pretty good' mode and should accept it. I'd make the same decision again.'

About eight weeks after his surgery, Arnold was back on the golf course. 'I was somewhat weak. I didn't have the strength that I felt I used to have. This is certainly a consequence of surgery, and you have to be ready for that. I'm still not totally at full strength, but I'm also getting older, so that may have something to do with it.'

Arnold Palmer has been through it. More importantly, he has emerged on the other side. Consequently, his opinion carries weight. And in his opinion, early detection is the key. 'Just get regular check-ups and PSAs and, if you're diagnosed, do everything you can to eradicate the disease. I think we are fortunate to have the best doctors in the world in this country [the US]. If you are not satisfied with the diagnosis and prognosis, then get a couple of opinions. But in the final analysis, you need to do what it takes to get rid of the cancer and get on with your life.'

Strong Feelings

Another high-profile US personality to have been touched by prostate cancer is former senator Bob Dole. He felt so strongly about the issue that he made a statement to the powerful Senate Appropriations Subcommittee on Labor, Health and Human Services.

His statement went as follows. 'Thank you for inviting me here this morning to discuss prostate cancer. It seems that just about every family in America has been touched in some way by cancer. My family has. And I have.

'Over eight years ago, I was diagnosed with prostate cancer. I was lucky to have had the disease diagnosed early and treated promptly through surgery. Eight years later, I am happy to say that I am cancer-free.

'Since the time of my diagnosis, I have tried to speak out as much as possible about the value and importance of early detection. I truly believe that early detection saved my life.

'The cancer was found when it was still contained within the prostate gland and when I had a variety of treatment options from which I had to choose.

'I will use this opportunity to say again: if you are a male over age forty, particularly if you have a family history [of prostate cancer], ask your doctor about getting a prostate check-up.

'People ask me how I can be so open about my own experience with prostate cancer. I must admit, when I first started speaking out about this disease, there were plenty of awkward moments. But then I decided that the alternative - silence - can be deadly.

'So when I am fortunate enough to be asked to testify before Congress on this issue, I do it.

'While my message of the importance of early detection is one that I will continue to deliver, I would like to take a moment to talk about treatment options.

'When I was diagnosed, I was basically given two options: surgery or radiation. That was it.

'I was told of the side effects of both, the risks of the procedures and the probability of cure. I have to admit, it was almost a toss-up. Both had side effects that sounded unpleasant, to say the least. But both had high rates of success. I chose surgery. And since I am cancer-free today, I of course believe I made the right decision.

'But every day there is a scientist looking for a cure for cancer, or looking for a new treatment option. And one of these days – I think in the not-so-distant future – there will be a cure. But the question is: will we recognise it when we see it?

'I think that is an important question for members of Congress and the administration to think about. Is our government prepared to take the steps that are necessary so that when new technology for treatment becomes available, patients with the disease can access it?

'One example is the proposed change in the reimbursement rate for an innovative prostate treatment known as brachytherapy. This therapy involves the implantation of radioactive seeds in the prostate directly. The seeds emit radiation that destroys cancer cells while minimising exposure to surrounding tissues. For some patients, this minimally invasive procedure, done on an outpatient basis, has been shown to treat some forms of prostate cancer.

'Currently, Medicare reimburses for this procedure. But if reimbursement is reduced, as is currently proposed, this type of technology will become less available to patients.

'As our health-care system continues to evolve and change, policymakers must encourage the adoption of innovative therapies. What's the point of science making advances every day if there is no way to deliver the technologies to patients who need them?'

Irish legislators would do well to heed his words.

21

There and Back Again

Our journey has taken us to Lisbon, Paris, Florence and America, but I have decided to come back to Listowel in an attempt to pull all the strands together. I travel by bus, to give myself time to read a few of John B.'s works, chief among which (for me) is *The Field*. I love the raw determination of the Bull McCabe and his single-minded focus on pursuing what he thinks is right; I love the barrenness of the Irish landscape depicted in the book; I love the rhythm of the language.

On the bus down to Market Square, I am surrounded by the music that is the Kerry accent. It puts me in mind of the time I met John B. himself, and the great friend-liness and good humour with which he greeted us; like stumbling across a long-lost friend.

There is a famous quote by John B. In a way, it sums up both his own determination and the funny slant he had on life. It came during a 'pep talk' to a local GAA team, and it went something like this: 'Now listen, lads, I'm not happy with our tackling. We're hurting them, but they keep getting up.'

You know, if anyone could have tackled this disease, it was him . . . provided he had been given the chance.

Listowel is a beautiful place. Set in around the banks of the glorious River Feale, it has earned the title 'The Literary Capital of Ireland'. And nestling in a corner of the town park is Ireland's only public monument to the millions who went to their death in the gas chambers of the Nazi concentration camps.

John B.'s pub is still there, just as I remember it. Winking at me with quaintness; seducing me with the promise of food and drink and rest.

I go in. Nobody knows me. Why would they? I order a pint and move away from everybody into the snug; the same snug in which we had the privilege of interviewing the great man.

Two Sides

As John B. might have said himself: there are two sides to every story. The story of prostate cancer is no different.

It's easy to make a case against the introduction of a screening programme, because . . . we have no screening programme. There you go, case made!

But what about the case for such a programme? Let's look at the evidence: prac-
tically every specialist I spoke with
agreed that if you look for something, you
have a better chance of finding it. They
agreed that prostate cancer is much the
same as any other cancer, in that if you
catch it early, you have a better chance
of a positive outcome.

Two of the leading Irish professors in
this area, John Armstrong and John
Fitzpatrick, have been advocates for
screening. Now, they would settle for a
dedicated Irish study to examine the fea-
sibility of a screening programme. People
who deal with this problem on a daily
basis, such as Ursula Courtney of ARC
House and Dr Sean Dunphy, are also in
favour of screening.

Professor Fred Stephens of the
University of Sydney, and author of one of
the most important texts on prostate cancer (*All About Prostate Cancer*), says:
'The earlier a patient seeks medical
attention for anything unusual or different, the more likely it will be that any
cancer will be detected at a curable
stage.'

Dr Patrick Walsh of the Johns Hopkins
Hospital in the US says: 'Since screening
came in, fewer men present with cancer
that has spread. More men present with
curable disease.'

Dr Andrew von Eschenback of the
National Cancer Institute in the US says:
'Our best weapon today to deal with

cancer is to be able to find it early, at a time when we can still effectively apply treatment.'

Dr Liam Twomey, former health spokesperson for Fine Gael, is in favour of all forms of screening and has drafted a policy document on the issue.

Liz McManus, the Labour Party's spokesperson on health, says: 'I accept fully that screening for prostate cancer should be implemented.'

American politicians, including Rudy Giuliani, Colin Powell and Bob Dole, are strong supporters of prostate screening.

They can't all be wrong. Can they?

Outside, a light rain is beginning to brush my face, and the first strands of evening darkness are descending softly on the streets of Listowel.

I breathe in deeply. There is a vague hint of turf in the air.

I feel a weight lift from me. The question has been asked.

There you go, John B. I said I'd ask the question for you. Now, let's see if we can get some real answers.

As I walk to my bus, a little woman bundled up in a great coat and festooned with shopping bags comes towards me.

I smile at her.

'Hello,' she says, smiling back. 'Are you well?'

'Never better,' I say. 'Never better.'

Epilogue

One of the big arguments against introducing a prostate screening programme has always been the lack of a major screening study. Now, a number of those 'major studies' have just concluded, and they have found that PSA screening does, in fact, cut mortality from prostate cancer.

It's worth repeating: PSA screening cuts mortality.

One such study was carried out in Québec, Canada. It involved tens of thousands of men and lasted a full eleven years. The researchers found a 'strongly positive and highly significant' relationship between the rate of PSA testing and a reduction in deaths from prostate cancer.

They further found that a 10 percent increase in the rate of PSA testing more than doubled the annual reduction in mortality from prostate cancer.

The study leader was Dr Bernard Candas, who plies his trade at the Oncology and Molecular Endocrinology Research Centre in Laval, Québec.

He said: 'Metastatic prostate cancer should be avoidable through screening. So, more and more patients should be treated at an early stage.'

There are now a significant number of population-based studies showing positive outcomes in relation to prostate-cancer prevention and early intervention. Here are just two more to give you a flavour of the kind of research scientists involved in the area of the prostate are engaged in:

A major population-based screening programme concluded in the Iranian city of Tehran in 2004. The study ran for nine years and 3,670 men over the age of forty were included in it. They were all checked by PSA-based screening and were all invited to have a DRE. The Iranian doctors found that, in all, 138 of the men had prostate cancer and many more had elevated PSA readings, which warranted further investigation. The conclusion, according to the Iranian medical authorities, is: 'PSA-based screening (with low PSA cut-off values) *increases the detection rate* of clinically significant, organ-confined and potentially curable prostate cancer.'

In Sahlgrenska University Hospital in Sweden, a major population-based screening programme concluded recently. They looked at almost 10,000 men in their fifties and sixties. Men with a PSA reading of above 3.0 ng/ml were invited for further investigation. Altogether, 145

cancers were detected. The Swedes concluded that 'PSA screening detected
early-stage, low-grade prostate cancer'.

The message would appear to be simple:
based on these evidence-based studies,
screening saves lives!

APPENDICES

A question of prostate cancer

§ Do you sometimes pass urine when you don't expect to?

§ Do you pass urine three or more times during the night?

§ Are you bursting to go and then find that you barely produce a trickle?

§ Do you strain to pass urine, or does it take a long time to start?

§ When you pass urine, are you always stopping and starting?

§ Do you have any discomfort, such as pain or a burning sensation, when you pass urine?

§ Does your bladder still feel full after you've finished?

§ Is there any dribbling after you've stopped?

§ Have you ever seen blood in your urine?

Some of the main treatment options

for prostate cancer

Radical prostatectomy

This is a surgical procedure designed to remove the entire prostate gland. The surgeon will also target the lymph nodes, located close to the prostate, to reduce the risk of cancer spread. The main advantage of this approach is that once the surgeon goes in, all of the cancerous cells can be removed in one fell swoop. As with any surgery, there are a number of potential complications: some patients experience substantial loss of blood during the procedure, and the main side-effect risk factors are incontinence and impotence. The latest figures show, however, that incontinence following the procedure is rare and, if the surgeon is very careful, the nerves that help with sexual function can be preserved, so erectile dysfunction is also unlikely to be a long-term problem. The stay in hospital for this procedure is normally between two and three days, depending on the person's general state of health.

Radiation therapy

Radiation therapy can be administered via a machine or by means of implantation into the prostate gland itself. Both methods are roughly equally effective, but there are a number of options that the patient has to weigh up. Radiation administered via a machine (known as 'beam-radiation therapy') is extremely time-consuming. It is usually given five days a week over a seven-week period. Radiation implants go by the name 'brachytherapy' or 'seed therapy'. Essentially, radioactive pellets are injected into the prostate gland. The main advantage of seed therapy is that it can be done in just one hospital visit. Doctors acknowledge that there is a degree of hit-and-miss surrounding the radiation approach: because the prostate gland and the lymph nodes are not being removed, it is difficult to gauge the level of cancer spread.

Hormone therapy

Androgens are the target here. Androgens, which include testosterone, are produced mainly in the testicles. The problem is that these hormones help the tumour to grow in the prostate. Hormone therapy is usually the course of action adopted once the cancer has spread beyond the prostate and into surrounding organs. The good news is that, once the testosterone has been chased from the body, the prostate cancer usually shrinks. Hormone therapy is usually indicated for up to two years. Once it has been stopped, the cancer can reappear.

Prostate websites

www.cancer.ie

This is the Irish Cancer Society's official website. It contains up-to-the-minute news and information on issues affecting prostate cancer.

www.irishhealth.com

A dedicated Irish health website, which contains news, views and research findings on prostate cancer. Well written. A valuable resource if you want to stay right up to date with what is happening in Irish health.

www.cancerhelpo.org.uk

This site was set up to allow people to share stories, images and thoughts on dealing with prostate cancer.

www.prostatecancerfoundation.org

This site is a very user-friendly resource. It contains all the basic information on dealing with prostate cancer. It has videos on the subject, current articles and books, as well as tips from the experts. Highly recommended.

www.prostate-cancer.org.uk

This site is designed as a forum for people with prostate cancer to share their thoughts on how best the condition should be managed. It dubs itself 'Prostate Cancer Voices' and it lives up to its billing.

www.cancerscreening.nhs.uk

This site addresses more of the issues surrounding screening and, while not advocating it, it does contain valuable information for men considering a PSA test.

www.prostate-cancer-research.org.uk

This site is the home of the Prostate Cancer Research Centre in the UK, which carries out research into the condition. A good resource for keeping up to date on the very latest studies.

www.urosource.com

An international website containing all the latest research-based studies on the management of prostate cancer.

Further Reading

Joel Nathan, *What To Do When They Say It's Cancer: A Survivor's Guide* (1998)

Eckhart Tolle, *The Power of Now* (1998)

Ted Kaptchuk, *The Web That Has No Weaver* (2000)

Fred Stephens, *All About Prostate Cancer* (2000)

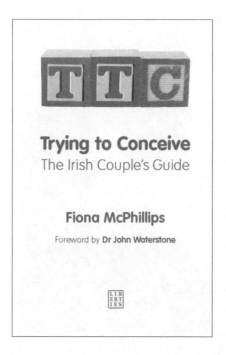

TTC

TRYING TO CONCEIVE: THE IRISH COUPLE'S GUIDE

€16.99 | 978–1–905483–36–5

The essential guide for couples dealing with problems relating to infertility. The medical causes of male and female factor infertility are discussed, and advice on ways of increasing fertility is provided. Includes comprehensive information on fertility clinics and related services and organisations across the island of Ireland.

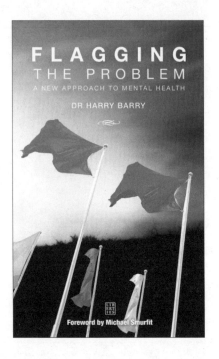

FLAGGING THE PROBLEM

A NEW APPROACH TO MENTAL HEALTH

€19.99 | 978–1–905483–18–1

The best-selling book presenting a ground-breaking approach
to mental health using a unique, flag-based system, from
respected GP and board member of Aware. Includes practical
information on helping friends and family members who may
be suffering from depression or other forms of
mental ill-health.